He

This series introduces a wide range of healing techniques that can be used either independently or as a complement to traditional medical treatment. Most of the techniques included in the series can be learnt and practised alone, and each encourages a degree of self-reliance, offering the tools needed to achieve and maintain an optimum state of health.

Each title opens with information on the history and principles of the technique and goes on to offer practical and straightforward guidance on ways in which it can be applied, with diagrams and case studies where appropriate. Please note that readers are advised to seek professional guidance for serious ailments, and to make use of the list of practitioners for further guidance. Many of the techniques in this series are taught in workshops and adult education classes; all of the titles are written by professional practitioners with many years of experience and proven track records.

AVAILABLE IN THIS SERIES

Healing with Colour — Helen Graham
Healing with Herbs — Judith Hoad
Healing with Meditation — Doriel Hall
Healing with Osteopathy — Peta Sneddon and
    Paolo Coseschi
Healing with Reflexology — Rosalind Oxenford

FORTHCOMING TITLES IN THIS SERIES

Healing with Ayurveda
Healing with Chinese Medicine
Healing with Crystals
Healing with Essential Oils
Healing with Feng Shui
Healing with Flower Essences
Healing with Nutritional Therapy
Healing with Shiatsu

Healing with Homeopathy

PETER CHAPPELL AND DAVID ANDREWS

Gill & Macmillan

Gill & Macmillan Ltd
Goldenbridge
Dublin 8
with associated companies throughout the world
© Peter Chappell and David Andrews 1996
0 7171 2421 5
Series editor: Tessa Strickland
Series copy editor: Pamela Dix
Index compiled by Helen Litton
Print origination by Typeform Repro Ltd, Dublin
Printed by ColourBooks Ltd, Dublin

A catalogue record is available for this book from the
British Library.

1 3 5 4 2

Contents

Acknowledgments

From Peter Chappell I would like to thank all my patients and students across Europe for their support of my learning through teaching, and especially those patients who have allowed me to publish their cases in detail. I thank Bill Gray especially for his *Thuja* remedy picture, Rajan Sankaran for his inspiration, and David Andrews for effectively co-writing this book. The best bits are mine, the mistakes are his ...

From David Andrews I would like especially to thank Rosalind Oxenford for her wisdom and support, and for putting Peter Chappell and me together to produce this book. And a big 'thank you' to Peter for teaching me so much about this wonderful subject. As for the mistakes ...

CHAPTER ONE

Why Homeopathy?

In recent years, an increasing number of people in the western world have come to recognise the benefits of the so-called complementary medicines, such as herbalism, acupuncture, osteopathy and reflexology. Most of these therapies have their roots deep in history, and have in some cases been practised for thousands of years. All have one thing in common: they work on the basis of treating the person in a holistic way. This means that the whole person, body, mind and soul, is treated — not just the symptoms showing on the surface.

During and after the Second World War, with the arrival of modern surgery, immunology and antibiotics, people put their complete confidence into symptomatic (conventional) medicine. However, an increasing interest in holistic medicine can be seen as a further evolution in thinking about health and disease.

Homeopathy is a new system of medicine compared with the other holistic systems and conventional medicine. However, homeopathy has been widely adopted by doctors and patients world-wide because its principles and practices are in line with the ancient systems of healing — and because it works so well. Simply put, it makes you feel good as well as healthy.

Homeopathy is available throughout Europe, North and South America, India and more than seventy other countries.

> Homeopathy treats the whole person, finding and
> treating the root cause of disease rather than
> suppressing its symptoms.

Homeopaths believe that there exists within everyone
an intelligent energy that maintains the balance in your
body, mind and emotions and controls the ability to heal
and maintain the organism. This is called the vital force, a
concept common in cultures throughout the world. In
acupuncture it is called *chi*, and in Indian culture it is
referred to as *prana*. Although this vital force cannot be
seen and is not yet recognised by science, its presence is
everywhere apparent. It's just that its presence is not
recognised for what it is. All medical students are taught
precisely how the body functions — what the liver,
kidneys, lungs etc. do — and they gain in-depth
knowledge of the mechanisms and functions of the human
body. They know that once these functions cease to
operate, then the body can be considered dead; yet do they
understand the real difference between an alive and a dead
body? What is behind the living data they measure? What
drives it?

To a homeopath, illness is a fundamental imbalance
occurring at a deep level within a person — this
imbalance is the root cause of disease. Symptoms show the
homeopath what remedy to use to help the body's own
natural defences.

As well as the physical symptoms, the homeopath will
also take into account the emotional state and experiences
that go to make up the picture of the whole person that is
his patient (see Chapter Nine, 'Case Studies'). For example,
it may be significant that you wake up at 3 a.m. each

morning; that you have sweaty feet; that you lost a parent at a young age; that you have a poor relationship with a parent or sibling. The more complete the picture, the more accurately the homeopath can prescribe.

> Homeopathy works *with* rather than *against* the body, stimulating its own powerful natural defence mechanisms and healing processes.

HOMEOPATHIC REMEDIES

Homeopathic remedies are drawn from nature — from minerals and metals, from plants and animals, from human diseases and now, in the nuclear age, from radiation sources. New remedies are created by a well defined systematic process, using experimentation (called proving) on human volunteers that gives the basic information homeopaths use to prescribe for their patients. The remedies are made by a repetitive diluting and shaking process called potentisation. The final product can be 'sugar of milk' pills soaked and dried as tablets, or a liquid. One pill at a time is put under the tongue — this is one dose.

Without harming them, the healing energies of living creatures such as eagles, lions, dolphins and scorpions are now being introduced into homeopathic practice, with long-used ones of snakes, fish and spiders. Where available the animal's milk is potentised; in the case of the eagle, the blood on a feather that came out of the bird by accident has been used.

Every homeopathic remedy has its own picture, and represents a particular condition and state of mind. Each person at a given time also has a picture which represents and reflects the way he or she feels, acts and thinks about him or herself and the environment.

A well-chosen homeopathic remedy can reverse most diseases of an internal origin at the outset, the rate of progress depending on the amount of pathological damage that has occurred. It also removes predispositions towards disease. It is particularly valuable in treating diseases in their formative stages, before a physical diagnosis can be made, so that health can be restored while it is still easily possible.

Homeopathy aims to match the remedy to the person. For example, *Aurum metallicum* (gold) is described in the homeopathic *Materia Medica* (the reference book which lists the characteristics and use of all the remedies) in this way: 'Gold makes a profound impression on the mind, producing acute mental depression, hopelessness and loss of love of life ...' (from its effects on healthy people); 'For the ill-effects of grief, fright, anger, disappointed love, contradiction, reserved displeasure, prolonged anxiety, unusual responsibility ...' (from clinical experience). *Aurum metallicum* can be helpful for people who are chronic alcoholics, deeply depressed, suicidal, or have lost the will to live. Their condition may also show as physical symptoms such as headaches, heart palpitations, acne, arthritis and swollen glands.

> By understanding the complete picture of a patient, the homeopath is able to treat mind, body and spirit simultaneously, achieving deep, long-term curative action.

GREEN MEDICINE

Homeopathic remedies are produced from naturally occurring substances, without causing damage to the environment. Quantities of substances required to make remedies are so small that the sources of these substances — plants, trees, minerals and animals — are easily sustainable.

Provings of these substances are made on healthy people who benefit, rather than on laboratory animals who suffer and die. As homeopathy is low-tech, there is no need for laboratories to engage in long-term research and development, or the involvement of multinational drug companies. Anybody with the right knowledge and care can potentise a substance and produce a remedy. As homeopathic remedies are safe and have no side-effects, there is no need for expensive testing and trials.

In addition, the average cost of a remedy — if you buy the minimum quantity of pills, and use one pill very occasionally as needed — is 15p. Compare this to a minimum prescription charge in the UK of around £5 per medicine. Given that you may be on two or three different drugs — one for pain, one for constipation caused by the painkillers and one for depression – the difference in cost could easily be one hundred times the amount spent on a homeopathic remedy for an equivalent period. The potentially high cost, both in personal terms and to your local health authority, may also be a waste of resources. The application of homeopathy in the developing nations who cannot afford 'western' medicine, and who have serious disease and public health problems, could have a profound effect on their national well-being as well as on their balance of payments. Homeopathy is safe, non-political, non-dogmatic, universal and cheap, and has many strong and influential supporters around the world.

An interesting example of how much homeopathy can offer can be found in Belarus, a European country with a population of ten million people. Belarus received seventy per cent of the radiation from the Chernobyl nuclear power disaster. Ninety-two per cent of the children there are sick, and cancer has increased one hundred fold. Treating these cancers is clearly a priority, and western aid has poured in to help.

However, for the two million children who are suffering from a variety of ailments such as growth retardation, frequent high fevers and herpes, but who do not have cancer, conventional medicine can offer little. By comparison, for these children homeopathy can and does offer proven results. It is also easily affordable in a country where orthodox medicines can cost a week's wages.

CHAPTER TWO

The History and Principles of Homeopathy

SAMUEL HAHNEMANN

One hundred and eighty-five years ago a revolutionary new form of medicine was launched into the world with the publication of Samuel Hahnemann's book *The Organon of the Rational Art of Healing.* The curative powers of this new medicine were, over the ensuing years, to be shown to have a beneficial effect on victims of the terrible epidemics of cholera, typhoid, yellow fever and scarlet fever that were to sweep through Europe and the United States, as well as on many forms of chronic disease.

Born the son of a porcelain painter on 10 April 1755, Samuel Hahnemann grew up in the town of Meissen in south-west Germany. He was a thin, delicate boy with a fair complexion and clear blue eyes. The Seven Years' War ran from 1756 to 1763, and consequently Hahnemann's childhood was marked by hardship, danger and restricted travel. As his parents were of limited financial means, he was educated by them at home during his early years, which gave him a grounding in broad general knowledge. Taught by his father never to learn or listen passively but to question everything, Hahnemann is said to have had the 'highest standards of moral behaviour'. He later attended the town elementary school, until the age of fifteen. This education was interrupted by the family's need for him to earn money, and he was often away from school — sometimes for up to a year at a time. However, he showed

a particular aptitude for languages, and he developed a
strong relationship with his teacher, Magister Johann
Muller, who also gave him extra lessons in Greek, Latin
and German.

In 1771, Hahnemann became a pupil at the Prince's
Grammar School, where Johann Muller had moved to
become Rector. During the following four years their
relationship developed into a lasting friendship, and with
Muller's guidance Hahnemann developed his skills in
languages, mathematics, geometry and botany.

In 1775, at the age of twenty, Hahnemann entered the
University of Leipzig — a university with a reputation as
a centre of culture and learning throughout Europe — to
study medicine. During his time at Leipzig he maintained
his meagre existence by teaching German and French and
translating Greek and English into German. Hahnemann
was disappointed in the lectures he received, finding that
he could often acquire more knowledge from selected
medical textbooks. 'I studied privately all the time, reading
always the best that was available and only as much as I
could assimilate ... I attended only such lectures as I
considered useful.' The lack of practical facilities for
medical study — there was no hospital or clinic available
— increased his frustration.

Hahnemann decided, late in 1776, to leave Leipzig for
Vienna. There he obtained the practical medical training he
needed under the tuition of Dr Quarin at the General
Hospital. At that time he also began to question the lack of
hygiene and compassion, the practices of blood-letting and
the use of leeches and nostrums (dubious patent medicines)
that he found in contemporary medical practice. Thus were
planted the seeds of discontent that were to germinate into
a new science of medical practice. Hahnemann eventually

completed his medical studies at the University of
Erlangen, and was awarded the degree of Doctor of
Medicine in August 1779, at the age of twenty-four.

Several years of medical practice were to follow,
during which time his disillusionment with the
conventional approach to medicine increased. At the same
time, Hahnemann studied chemistry, as well as translating
and reviewing many books, which led to the writing of his
own works on chemistry and medicine. He then gave up
medical practice in disgust in order to continue his own
private studies, whilst making a meagre living with his
literary work.

HOMEOPATHIC PRINCIPLES

Homeopathy has a number of core principles from which
a set of practices naturally follow. By applying these in a
comprehensive way, as an art and as a science, a deeply
curative healing process emerges.

SIMILIA SIMILIBUS CURENTUR — 'LET LIKE BE CURED WITH LIKE'

One of the works Hahnemann translated included *A
Treatise on Materia Medica* by Dr William Cullen, a leading
teacher, physician and chemist in Edinburgh. Cullen
devoted twenty pages of his book to the therapeutic
indications of Peruvian Bark (the source of quinine).
Hahnemann's enquiring mind was dissatisfied with
Cullen's explanation that the success of Peruvian Bark in
treating malaria lay in its bitterness. In order to further his
knowledge, Hahnemann undertook an unprecedented
experiment: he took a series of doses of Peruvian Bark
himself, and recorded the effects of a medicine on a
healthy person.

He wrote, 'Peruvian Bark, which is used as a remedy

for intermittent fever, acts because it can produce
symptoms similar to those of intermittent fever in healthy
people.' This proving of the drug was the start of important
research, and became one of the first principles of his new
method of treatment — homeopathy.

Hahnemann's observations opened up a revolutionary
new understanding of the nature of symptoms. He learned
that symptoms were the body's positive response to a
variety of stress experiences, rather than unhealthy
responses that needed to be treated, suppressed or
controlled. Symptoms were the body's efforts to heal itself.

> Rather than suppressing symptoms, treatment should
> stimulate the body's defences to complete the curative
> process.

Hahnemann's discovery attracted many other physicians, in
addition to much criticism from the medical
establishment. Over the years, his announcements and
books shook the medical world — exciting the public too
— but arousing tremendous opposition. This opposition
to his ideas became a theme in Hahnemann's life.

Hahnemann and like-minded colleagues began to
experiment on themselves by taking different remedies,
keeping detailed records of the symptoms produced by
each of them. They began to notice that these symptom
pictures were similar to those produced by illnesses for
which cures had been sought by medical science for many
years. The medicines were then tried on so-called
incurables, who were cured by the remedies when they
were prescribed according to this principle. This
experimental process, by which symptoms are created in a
healthy person, Hahnemann called provings.

POTENTISATION

In 1810 Hahnemann's *The Organon of the Rational Art of Healing* was published. The result of twenty years of arduous and difficult experimentation and observation, the book set out his principles of homeopathy and described his experiments with different strengths of remedies. He was aware that some of the substances were highly toxic in their concentrated form, and he discovered how to reduce the size of the dose, in order to eliminate the toxic effects without losing the healing qualities — a stroke of real genius. He achieved this by what is known as potentisation — the sequential dilution of the substance, along with a violent shaking of each dilution. The number of dilutions plus shakings — called succussions — he called the 'potency'; the first centesimal potency (1c) was a dilution of one part of the decimal potency to 99 parts water plus succusion. Repeating this three times produces the 3c potency; six times the 6c potency, and so on. The potency of the homeopathic remedies obtainable in most health food shops and chemists is 6c.

The LM1 potency is produced by taking 3c as above and diluting it 50,000 to one, and LM2 by another such dilution, and so on. The succussions are very important, as without them the diluted liquids lose all healing activity. Why this process works is still a mystery, but it can be measured and the effects are dramatically to be seen by use.

This was an astounding discovery. Clearly to scientists it is not logical that a substance diluted to one part in 100,000 or more can act to cure disease quickly, permanently and without side-effects. So how does it work? Science has shown that molecules show a constant movement, known as Brownian Motion. All molecules and

atoms are composed of energy, which can be measured
electromagnetically. J. Benveniste, a French research
scientist funded by his own government, reported in a
paper published in the scientific journal *Nature* in 1988
that he had found and measured electrically detectable
patterns in homeopathically prepared substances. It appears
that a remedy is effective when its electromagnetic field
resonates with or matches that of the disturbed or 'dis-
eased' vital force of the body. The resonance stimulates the
healing process.

Efforts were made by the medical and scientific
establishments to discredit Benveniste and his work
because it upset their belief system — how could such
substances have any effect? Benveniste's laboratory
practices and experiments were repeated around the
world, but were still questioned by other scientists. His
funding was withdrawn, and Benveniste lost his reputation
and ability to work because he had dared to question
established views.

THE HOLISTIC PRINCIPLE

A core principle that Hahnemann developed within
homeopathy related to holism, which he called 'the totality
of symptoms'. By this he meant that what is wrong with
someone is not merely one or two symptoms or a
diagnosis, but the whole disturbance in mind and body
taking in the widest possible view of life — what today
homeopaths call the maximum totality. This takes into
account the attitude, inner thoughts, outer expression, diet
and climate, relationships, work and creativity, sleeping,
dreams and fantasies, ambitions, will, determination, love,
sex, spirituality, emotions, current problems and problems
from conception onwards, as well as the state and nature of

the country the patient lives in.

Homeopaths also concentrate on the way a patient faces the challenges of life, the person's own unique responses. In this way they capture the core image of the inner energy that is stuck, the core pattern of malfunctioning, the deepest inner trauma, and bring about a profound cure of mind and matter so that the person comes to be more fully in the present time, and lives more in harmony with his or her inner spirit.

HERING'S LAWS OF CURE

Constantine Hering, a German homeopath who emigrated to the United States in the 1830s, is thought of as the father of American homeopathy. He formulated three general principles of the homeopathic healing process.

Hering states that the curing process progresses from the deepest levels of the organism — the mental and emotional — through the vital organs to the external parts such as skin and extremities. A cure is in progress when a person's psychological symptoms improve. As the healing moves outwards, the physical symptoms will also improve; the outermost symptoms — the skin for example — will be the last to heal. Healing progresses from the upper parts of the body to the lower, and from the vital organs to less important ones — from lungs to nose, from heart to skin, for example.

Conversely, if physical symptoms improve but the patient's psychological state worsens, then his or her state of health is said to be regressing.

Hering also states that as symptoms re-appear or disappear, they do so in reverse chronological order of appearance. These returning symptoms, in a chronic case, may be symptoms that patients re-experience from illnesses suffered years or even decades ago. They tend to pass quickly, without the intensity of the original illness.

As the symptoms change, it is common for a patient to experience a worsening of current complaints. This is a welcome sign that healing is in progress — as long as there is a corresponding improvement on a deeper level.

In the light of modern psychology, I would express this somewhat differently. (The following does not apply to genetic disease, or disease which is inherited or related to adverse external circumstances.) Disease which is rooted in unresolved trauma is stored up internally as emotional conflict, and manifests as blocked energy through tension, stresses, stiffness and pain; all forms of mental and physical illness — down to the cell level — will unravel in the reverse way to its formation process. The most recent traumas of a similar type will be released first, and the earliest trauma last.

In particular, as the trauma is released by the activation of a healing intervention (such as a homeopathic remedy) the vital energy flows again and dissolves the block. A temporary replay of the old trauma will result in the appropriate emotion — anger, fear, grief, loss — about past events. If these are expressed directly there will be no physical effect, but if they are repressed according to the normal pattern — by far the most likely option — then they will regenerate temporarily the old patterns of illness, which homeopaths call the aggravation.

INHERITED DISEASE IN HOMEOPATHY
Hahnemann wrote extensively about miasms, his label for inherited disease patterns. Today we would articulate these patterns more clearly as the result of both inherited

emotional trauma and the continuing effects of inherited disease. (See Chapter Seven, 'Chronic Diseases'.)

HOMEOPATHY AND MODERN SCIENCE

We are in an era of radical scientific change. The fundamentals of science over the last 2,000 years, formatted on the logic of Aristotle, are being revised in favour of a deeper and more profound understanding of the universe. Chaos theory — stating that small changes in the physical world can over time have unpredictable and possibly major consequences — is causing a revolution in our understanding of energy patterns; homeopathic principles are underpinned by chaos theory. A homeopathic remedy is like a chaos 'strange attractor' energy pattern.

Because of chaos theory, the idea that an individual's state of health should be indicated by steady measurements like blood pressure has been rejected in favour of variability according to circumstances. In medical terms, this means a healthy heart has a variable rate, and its variability is a measure of health. Conventional drugs for 'bad hearts' stabilise the heart rate in a way that nature may not have intended. Other orthodox medical drugs have the same basic problem. For example, cortisone does not cure asthma or eczema; it instead suppresses the effects temporarily. Homeopathy and chaos theory show that this comes with the penalty of a reduction in overall health and vitality, taking the person in a potentially deathly direction.

Fuzzy maths, a revolution in the field of maths, has shown that the whole is more than the sum of the parts, and not as Descartes said, 'just equal to the parts'. Whereas conventional medicine still believes that we are merely flesh and bones, homeopathy sees a person as a spirit-like energy, mobilising the body with a vitality that works through our mind/body into activity and expression.

Quantum physics has shown that mind and matter occur inseparably together, as two aspects of the same energy.

These comparatively recent changes in scientific thought confirm the findings of Samuel Hahnemann — two centuries later. Homeopathy is therefore being substantiated by every major scientific advance, as well as by specific research including double-blind controlled trials.

HOMEOPATHY AND PSYCHOLOGY

Hahnemann lived well before Freud and Jung, so his awareness of particular psychological issues, though profound, was not articulated with the depth of understanding we are familiar with today. He did, however, cite emotional trauma as the major influence on ill health. The fruits of psychotherapeutic understanding are now being integrated into homeopathic processes, offering a better understanding of what is to be cured.

> Homeopathy links mind and body as one inseparable energy.

SAMUEL HAHNEMANN'S LATER LIFE

Hahnemann eventually received support from a local duke, away from conflict and the opposition of the medical profession, and further developed his research, theories, principles and practices. He said, 'In a peaceful environment, away from all the hostility, there was time to apply my mind to some of the theoretical questions which had been troubling me for some time, about the causes of disease, the regulatory force within the organism ...'

At the age of eighty, Hahnemann was winding down his life — his wife was dead, his daughters were looking after him — when a remarkable thing happened. A thirty-five-year-old Parisian woman called Melanie was so excited by Hahnemann's books that she travelled across Europe to visit him. They fell in love, and the old man was rejuvenated. They moved to Paris, where they soon began to treat people from the old and new worlds. Homeopathy took off amongst royalty and the rich and prosperous, spreading overseas, making particular inroads into America among doctors and other practitioners and as a self-help system. By 1900, around ten per cent of medicine in America had become homeopathic.

Hahnemann died on 2 July 1843, aged eighty-eight. His grave is in Père Lachaise cemetery in Paris, and there are also monuments to him in Washington D.C. and elsewhere. Melanie Hahnemann continued to practise, and was the first woman homeopath without an orthodox medical background. Hahnemann's followers included both doctors and non-doctors. The leading figures in homeopathy world-wide today include many people who have never had orthodox medical training.

THE SUPPRESSION OF HOMEOPATHY

Medical opposition to homeopathy unfortunately grew rapidly at the beginning of the twentieth century, despite considerable support for Hahnemann's work. This, combined with expectations that science would eliminate disease, led to homeopathy being effectively put on the back burner of medicine by 1920. By the 1960s, only a few stalwarts remained. However, as world consciousness moved to greener pastures, holistic thinking was validated by medical and scientific research. Homeopathy, along with other forms of alternative, holistic medicine, has again moved into the ascendancy. It seems likely that this time holistic medical approaches will become the front-line systems in a cohesive, balanced health creation rather than a disease-management health care system.

CHAPTER THREE

Theory into Practice

THE HOLISTIC APPROACH AND
UNDERSTANDING THE CAUSES OF ILLNESS

In Chapter One I talked about the vital force that exists within us all and motivates and energises our psyche and bodily functions. Our experiences in life affect this vital force, so the way we *feel* is in reality our state of health at any given time.

The word 'psychosomatic' derives from two Greek words *psyche* (soul or mind), and *soma* (body). We exist in our minds and in our bodies simultaneously. And mind and body can never be separate, even for a microsecond. We are all psychosomatic beings. For example, all of us from time to time suffer from anxiety and worry — and some forms of worry are more 'serious' than others. Worry begins in the mind, but it resonates in the body as well — we often feel it in our tummies.

Most people have worries about exams before sitting them, but some people suffer severe anxiety. The somatic side of this may manifest as sleeplessness, nausea, stomach cramps, headaches or — in extreme cases — the person may become so unwell that he cannot attend the examination. He may believe he has food poisoning, because the symptoms are diarrhoea and vomiting. What has happened is that the worry that began in the mind has manifested as dramatic symptoms (diarrhoea and vomiting that has been dismissed as food poisoning).

> Homeopaths believe that there is no such thing as an
> illness — only ill people.

Much illness has a psychologically-based root cause, even
cancer. How is it that in a room full of people
contaminated with, say, influenza not everybody will
'catch' (attract) the disease? The people that get the disease
are in some way vulnerable at the outset to the invasion of
the virus, as their immune system is compromised. This is
often the result of trauma — recent or remote —
combined with inherited weaknesses from past diseases in
the family.

WHAT IS THE ROOT CAUSE OF DISEASE?

The homeopath's job is to find the root cause of disease in
an individual, and to treat it accordingly to bring about a
long-term and profound cure. But this only works if the
homeopath can find out what the 'disease' pattern is and
match it precisely to the correct remedy. For this to
happen, the homeopath will 'take the case', which involves
a long (usually one to two hours) and careful interview
with the patient. It helps if the patient is a willing
participant, or has a willing parent or carer, and if she is
honest, truthful and open about everything, whether she
believes it to be relevant or not. However, we all have
'blind spots', tell lies or don't want to talk about
something, so it is up to the homeopath to use all his or
her skills to observe, perceive and collect the relevant
information. Questions need to be wide open, so that they
do not lead the patient into saying what she thinks the
homeopath wants to hear.

  The homeopath needs to give the patient the space

and freedom to communicate who she really is, and what deeply held beliefs have led her to be in the state of dis-ease that has bought her to the consulting room. He or she needs to be able to read all the signs and distinguish which of them are relevant to the case.

> The homeopath must be the unprejudiced observer, and have empathy, rather than sympathy, for the patient.

The homeopathic approach is to:
- understand the situation
- formulate the problem exactly
- pick the unique and characteristic signs and symptoms that represent the core problem
- select a remedy whose picture covers the core issue well.

And the cure naturally follows.

CASE ONE

Recently a father brought his eight-year-old daughter to see me. He reported that she was suffering from constipation (including ruptured haemorrhoids), and was anxious and introverted as well as having nightmares. The girl appeared in the consulting room to be a healthy, intelligent and sunny child. During the consultation it was difficult to balance what the father was telling me about his daughter (he was separated from her mother, and saw his daughter during weekends and holidays) and what I could learn from the girl herself.

I began to think that there was an abandonment issue going on inside her, caused by the break-up of her parents' relationship when she was three years old, and I felt that *Pulsatilla* was the right remedy for her. I gently asked the girl how she felt when she went home after the weekend with Dad. Tears welled up in her eyes.

Just before the end of the session, as I was looking something up in my *Materia Medica* and allowing space for anything else to emerge, her father said, 'I don't know if it's important, but she never has butter on her bread.' For me, this was the last piece of the jigsaw puzzle, proving conclusively that *Pulsatilla* was the correct remedy, and was highly effective. Pulsatilla people feel abandoned, weep easily, are averse to fat food — and particularly dislike butter. This illustrates how the space at the end of the consultation allowed the crucial detail about butter to emerge.

> Physical and psychological trauma weakens the vital force and lays the body open to attack.

CASE TWO

One patient who came to see me was a thirty-year-old man, with a burning pain in his stomach. He pointed to one spot (the beginnings of an ulcer). He seemed to be a workaholic, with two jobs and a habit of *rushing* from place to place. The man was very extrovert — even embarrassingly so — telling me intimate sexual indiscretions within minutes of arriving for the consultation. I wondered why he worked so hard, and by probing discovered that he *felt very alone*, and so surrounded himself with people and activity to hide this.

He had a *very sweet tooth, and loved salt*, a common but homeopathically useful combination. The man also had quite a number of fears — especially *claustrophobia* and a

fear of heights, as he gets the *impulse to jump*. He had a
naive sense of *generosity*, and liked to help others.

The words in italics add up to the homeopathic
remedy *Argentum nitricum*, which I prescribed and which
had a profound effect on the man. He left one job and
stopped rushing around so much; began having a social life
and found a girlfriend. After an initial worsening, the ulcer
pain improved and then disappeared. (I have often seen
this transition from childlike boy to adult after this
remedy.)

CHAPTER FOUR

Homeopathy and Self-Help

For ease of reference, we can group situations where homeopathy can be used for self-help into three categories: First Aid, Acute Illness and Emotional Trauma.

I recommend that you begin by trying out your skills on First Aid. After you have gained some knowledge and understanding of homeopathy, then you may try to treat acute illnesses. Emotional traumas need the help of a professional homeopath or more information, and you should not attempt to treat them without this.

> In homeopathy the only area of specifics — giving a remedy for a complaint or incident, not for the whole person — is First Aid.

Most people respond the same way in accidents and emergencies. In all other situations the homeopath considers a case and prescribes on the individual's unique reaction to the cause of a condition or disease.

FIRST AID REMEDIES

Unless otherwise indicated, the dose when a remedy is taken in tablet form is always 6c.

ARNICA (LEOPARD'S BANE) Bruises

No household (or handbag) should be without *Arnica*. I always carry some with me when I'm away from home, as it is so often the first remedy to take in the event of a physical accident with bruising. It works well with injuries of the soft parts of the body — the muscles and flesh.

For: shock, with bruising (see also *Bellis perennis*); bruising and sprains (see also *Ruta*); muscle-strain; bleeding; after surgery (take before and for a few days after); after strokes and cerebral accidents; concussion; dental extractions; loss of sight or hearing after head injury; bruises to the breast (see also *Conium*); tired muscles after exertion; childbirth, as it promotes delivery, relieves pains and helps to control haemorrhage.

The person needing *Arnica* is:

Worse from: touch, motion, damp cold.

Better from: lying down with head low.

Examples of using *Arnica*:

1   I was staying for the weekend with some friends. In the middle of the afternoon their six-year-old son was carried into the house by his elder brother. He was crying and screaming with pain and shock from having fallen on sharp gravel whilst running, and his legs were badly grazed. Within a few minutes of me giving him *Arnica* he had forgotten about his fall and was playing again. The next day there was no bruising visible, and the cuts were healing rapidly.

2   I was caught with one leg in the reins of a bolting horse, and dragged along on my back by this one leg for fifty yards or so. It became very obviously longer than the other! *Arnica* immediately took away the trauma (and osteopathy quickly put the structure right). *Arnica* is very useful before osteopathy or chiropractic manipulation for an injury to the structure — it takes away the trauma so the limb can then be re-aligned easily. Once again it speeds recovery.

3   I was involved in a car crash, being hit side on. I went unconscious from the impact on the side of my head. In hospital I took *Arnica*, then *Hypericum*, and I recovered quickly and completely, though it was a severe accident.

HYPERICUM (ST JOHN'S WORT) Injuries to Nerves and Spine

Hypericum is a remedy for injury, especially of the nerves and spine. Its hallmark is the sharp, shooting quality of the pains; they move up the limb from the wound.

For: lacerations (jagged cuts); crushed fingers and toes; injury to nerve-rich parts (tongue, teeth, eyes, genitalia, etc.); compound fractures; falls on the coccyx (tail-bone); pain in the coccyx following childbirth; injuries to any part of the spine; dental pain; phantom limb pain (suffered by amputees).

The person needing *Hypericum* is:

Worse from: damp, fog, cold, movement, touch.

Better from: bending head back, lying on front, rubbing.

LEDUM (MARSH TEA) Piercing Flesh Wounds

This is usually the remedy for such accidents as puncture wounds. It also prevents the sepsis in most of these types of injuries, and if given early enough in conjunction with *Hypericum* it can prevent tetanus. *Ledum* pills and tincture are a must for your homeopathic first aid kit. You can use the tincture, a few drops diluted in a little boiled water, to clean wounds, or in a poultice as a dressing. The tincture, used neat, is good for inflamed insect bites, especially those from fleas. *Ledum* is also a remedy for severe bruising with dark discoloration, where *Arnica* is not effective enough.

For: puncture wounds — splinters, stepping on nails, cat bites, etc.; sprains, especially in lower limbs, with marked bruising and effusion; purple discolorations and swelling; black eye from direct bruising; insect bites and stings; puncture wounds with suppuration; swelling or inflamed foot and ankle or lower leg where there is a tremendous desire to put feet in cold or even ice water.

The person needing *Ledum* is:

Worse from: heat, warm applications, night.

Better from: cold applications, ice, etc.

RUTA (RUE — BITTERWORT) **Sprains**

This remedy is especially useful for sports injuries and aches and pains caused by physical work such as gardening and labouring.

For: bruised muscles; torn or wrenched tendons; inflammation of the ligaments, knee and wrist joints; housemaid's knee; tennis elbow; bruises and kicks on the shin; RSI (repetitive strain injury); eye strain; eye stiffness caused by and worse from doing fine work; injuries to connective tissue, tendons and periosteum (outer covering of the bone); strains, sprains or twisting of joints resulting in a stiff, bruised pain.

The person needing *Ruta* is:

Worse from: cold air, stooping, exertion.

Better from: warmth, lying on back.

SYMPHYTUM (COMFREY) **Broken Bones**

Comfrey grows wild in some parts of the British Isles, and has been used by herbalists and physicians for centuries. Its old name — knitbone — makes it clear what it is for: it promotes healing in broken bones.

For: fractures, both acute and where there is non-union; injuries to the periosteum and bone with persisting pains long after the injury; injuries to the eyeball and

surrounding bone (orbital periosteum) caused by blunt
instruments (see also *Arnica* and *Ledum*).

Treatment for a broken bone: Give *Arnica* first, every one to
four hours, until the shock has passed (usually twenty-four
hours); then give *Ledum* to help reduce bruising, three
times a day (for around three to four days); then give
Symphytum three times a day until the bone is set and
repaired. You can also drink tea, made from Comfrey
leaves.

URTICA URENS (STINGING NETTLE) Burns

For: burns; relief of stinging nettle stings.

Treatment: If a blister has already formed, be careful not to
break it and apply *Urtica urens* locally. Add twenty drops of
tincture to a large cup of water and use the liquid to soak
a gauze, large enough to cover the whole area; cover with
lint, cotton wool and bandage.

Use this remedy in pill form to relieve the pain.
Repeat the dose whenever the pain returns.

For first degree and not too extensive second degree burns: Use
Urtica urens externally and internally.

For second degree burns: Use *Cantharis* or *Causticum*
internally for the burn pains where *Urtica urens* is not
sufficient; use *Calendula* lotion and ointment as the skin
begins to grow over the raw area. Use *Urtica urens*
ointment for stinging nettle stings.

You can make *Urtica urens* yourself from stinging
nettles. Pick some leaves, put in a pan with a cup of water;
simmer for five minutes; cool; soak a gauze in the mixture
and cover the burn.

CALENDULA OFFICINALIS (MARIGOLD) Cuts and Grazes

Calendula inhibits the growth of bacteria, can reverse the process of sepsis and infection and speed the healing process. Buy it as a tincture to dilute in water and as an ointment. Keep both in your first aid kit, as one may be more appropriate than the other, depending on the type of wound being treated. The ointment is very soothing, highly effective and quick to work. Use *Calendula* instead of antiseptics.

For: cleaning dirty wounds; when you change a dressing (tincture); healing all kinds of cuts, grazes, cracks, chapped hands and small septic spots (ointment).

HEPAR SULPH (CALCIUM SULPHIDE) Septic Wounds

This remedy will hasten suppuration in septic wounds filled with pus that are very sensitive to touch, and it takes away the acute pain.

For: septic wounds filled with pus that are too painful or difficult to clean.

The person needing *Hepar sulph* is:

Worse from: cold draughts, winter, lying on painful part.
Better from: heat, damp weather.

SILICEA

For: persistent abscesses.

PYROGEN

In sepsis this remedy is better than an antibiotic, and works more quickly too.

For: septic fever after childbirth when the placenta has been removed but part of it is left behind rotting; septic

wounds like cat bites leading to rosy red streaks going up
the arm or leg.

SECALE
For: frostbite and gangrene.

BELLIS PERENNIS (DAISY) Repeated Internal Bruising

This remedy is indicated in trauma, though less often than
Arnica, and is similar to *Arnica* in many respects. (If *Arnica*
often seems not to be helping a patient, then *Bellis perennis*
should be considered instead.)

For: internal bruising (baby's head in the womb pressing
on the sciatic nerves); sciatica; sprains; bruises (sore, bruised
sensations); lacerations or incisions where there is bleeding;
after surgery and bruising of the trunk of the body both
for the pain and to speed recovery.

The person needing *Bellis perennis* is:

Worse from: heat of bed or hot bath, chill.

Better from: continued motion, cold applications.

> First aid may also require bandages and surgical
> procedures. Attend a conventional first-aid course
> and/or buy a good self-help book to familiarise
> yourself with the correct procedures.

ACUTE ILLNESSES (ACUTES)

This section is about homeopathic remedies useful for
short-term illnesses that arise quickly from obvious outside
causes — called acute illnesses. There are, however, two
types of situation where there appears to be an acute
illness, and only one where the illness is truly acute. These
two situations need separating.

The most commonly understood acute is when you have 'caught' something: flu, a cold, a virus, a sore throat, a fever, a cough, food poisoning, a hangover, an allergic reaction, etc. In these cases there is a strong outside source of the problem.

However, there are many apparent acute illnesses which are not acutes at all, but outbreaks of an underlying condition. For example, some headaches, some allergic reactions, herpes, asthma attacks, epilepsy, diarrhoea without cause and recurring fever all have an inner cause. While the outbreak of these acute illnesses from an inner cause may be serious and need some form of immediate first aid (an asthma attack for example), the acute treatment and long-term cure needs professional homeopathic help.

I shall consider here only simple acute illnesses with obvious external causes, and not apparent acute illnesses resulting from an outbreak of a long-term internal illness.

REMEDY OPTIONS

Many people respond to external acute illnesses in line with their constitutional remedy, and any such illnesses they contract require remedies that relate to their constitution.

For example, Calcarea carbonicum people often have acute illnesses that may be cured with *Belladonna*; Natrum mur people have acutes that may be cured by *Bryonia* and *Ignatia*; Sulphur types have acutes that may be cured by *Arsenicum*; Silicea types have acutes that may be cured by *Pulsatilla*, etc. When you get a good result with a remedy, therefore, make a note of it.

However, while the above may be true, it is important to consider the symptoms with care, as they are the only true guide to the appropriate remedy.

REMEDIES FOR ACUTE ILLNESS

ACONITE (MONKSHOOD) Sudden Onset Acutes, Mental and Physical Shocks

This is a plant which grows high up in the mountains and relieves exposure to severe chill, or the response to a traumatic event such as witnessing a sudden death. This remedy is appropriate for acutes in which the symptoms begin within minutes or hours, not days, after the event (see *Gelsemium* and *Bryonia*).

Signs and Symptoms: illnesses that begin with a shock, a sudden chill or a sudden fright, and are accompanied by great fear of death; fever caused by chill or shock; croup (see below). In fever the face is hot and flushed or deadly pale, with a very anxious look; dry and burning (see *Belladonna*), yet chilly on the slightest motion, with thirst, restlessness, and chill alternating with heat. Throat red, dry, and constricted. Headaches hot, and could be from sunstroke. Any cough can be hoarse, dry and croupy. Croup is an infectious cough that can pass round the family one after the other; it has a dry stage, a wet stage, and a suffocative stage; worst time around midnight.

Treatment for croup: Aconite for the dry stage, *Hepar sulph* for the wet stage (when there is a lot of mucous in the lungs), and *Spongia* for the suffocative stage (when it is like breathing through a sponge).

AESCULUS HIPPOCASTANUM (HORSE CHESTNUT) Haemorrhoids

This remedy is good for piles, where after long and often useless straining to pass stools there is an intense pain in the anus for hours, and a full-up feeling.

Signs and Symptoms: piles (swollen veins in the anus); see also *Nux vomica* and *Sulphur*.

COLLINSONIA
Signs and Symptoms: piles in pregnancy.

HAMAMELIS
Signs and Symptoms: weight, rawness and burning in rectum, piles that protrude and bleed profusely; hard, knotted, swollen and painful veins.

ALLIUM CEPA (RED ONION) Hay Fever
Hay fever is only sometimes best treated as an acute. When you cut onions, they make your eyes itch and you produce tears — this remedy is for hay fever that produces similar symptoms. It is important in treating hay fever not to drive it in deeper. If you take any medicine — homeopathic or otherwise — and the hay fever symptoms get better but your chest, breathing or throat develop symptoms you did not previously have, then you are driving the problem deeper and you should stop taking the remedy immediately. Try something else, or consult a homeopath. New symptoms are a sign that the remedy is definitely wrong — they are not mere 'side-effects'.
Signs and Symptoms: hay fever which produces profuse but bland tears while nose discharge makes the skin red and burn; nose runs like a tap; aggravated by flowers.

Other remedies for hay fever include the following:

EUPHRASIA
Signs and Symptoms: hay fever and symptoms that include bland nose discharge; profuse tears; burning, red, itchy eyes, with intense blinking.

WYETHIA

Signs and Symptoms: hay fever and tremendous itching in nose, throat and palate; palate is scratched by the tongue.

ARUNDO

Signs and Symptoms: hay fever and symptoms including excess saliva.

ARUM TRIPHYLLUM

Signs and Symptoms: hay fever and very sore cracked lips and red around mouth with hoarseness; worse on right side.

SABADILLA

Signs and Symptoms: hay fever and symptoms including persistent, violent sneezing; worse from odours and perfumes.

SANGUINARIA

Signs and Symptoms: hay fever and symptoms including sensitivity to odour of flowers and pollens; right sided; burning.

The constitutional remedy, such as *Pulsatilla* or *Arsenicum,* is usually — though not always — best for hay fever; such a remedy will cure it for good if its basis is constitutional. This is the most satisfactory cure, and requires professional help.

ARSENICUM Food Poisoning

Arsenicum people have a fear of dying (but not as urgently as Aconite types) with intense restlessness, and are worse at 1 a.m. Whatever is wrong is likely to be burning which

unusually will be improved by heat; so an internal burning that is better from hot drinks, or a burning pain that is better from sitting on the radiator, is classic *Arsenicum*.
Signs and Symptoms: food poisoning; sudden great weakness from trivial causes; burning like fire; great anxiety about the seriousness of the complaint; very demanding of company and fresh air; gurgling in the food pipe (oesophagus) when drinking; diarrhoea with coldness, weakness, and possibly vomiting.
Dose: 200c potency, although frequent use of 6c will often suffice.

Other remedies for food poisoning include the following:

VERATRUM ALBUM
Signs and Symptoms: symptoms similar to above, but with greater intensity and less anguish.
Dose: 200c potency, although frequent use of 6c will often suffice.

CHINA AND CARBO VEG
(See page 37.)
Signs and Symptoms: pick-me-ups after food poisoning.

BELLADONNA (DEADLY NIGHTSHADE) High Fever
This is the number one high fever remedy.
Signs and Symptoms: high fever, where temperatures reach 40°C (104°F) with intense burning heat inside and out; earache when child cries out in sleep, is worse from noise and with a hot mouth and an inflamed, red throat, more right-sided; sunstroke, burning heat; bright red skin; dryness with no thirst or only rarely thirsty; some fear (less than Aconite people); throbbing, congestion; right-sided;

little or no sweat (maybe on forehead only); dilated pupils;
staring; delirium — even wildly delirious with
hallucinations; cold hands and feet with the rest burning
hot; over-sensitive to noise and light; generally worse at
3 p.m. and after midnight (bear in mind that fevers usually
peak in the evening and early part of the night, and last for
two days, and are a healthy sign that the self-healing ability
of the body is working).

Other remedies for high fever include the following:
STRAMONIUM / OPIUM
When high fever is accompanied by cold extremities and a
hot head the two above remedies are indicated. Use
Stramonium where there is less heat in the fever and more
spasms and delirium; use *Opium* when the pupils of the
eye are contracted.

BRYONIA (WILD HOPS) Pain Worse any Motion

A keynote indication for Bryonia people is that they hate
all motion when acutely ill, and do not wish to be
disturbed at all. These patients are easy to nurse because
they wish to be left alone. *Bryonia* is the best acute chest
remedy, whenever there is dryness of the mucous
membranes. These people need to drink a lot, with long
intervals between drinks, as even drinking disturbs them.
Signs and Symptoms: pleurisy (when the lung wall
lubricating fluid dries up); slow onset, mild fevers around
38.5°C (101°F); pain of broken bones (needs high
potency); after use of *Arnica* for joint injury if *Arnica* fails;
splitting headaches, better from closing the eyes (patient
holds the head); painful cough (patient holds the sore
part); sharp pain in the chest; generally worse at 9 p.m.;

worse from rising up, stooping, coughing, deep breathing, touch, eating, talking; better lying on painful part and bandaged, as this restricts movement.

CARBO VEG

This remedy is commonly known as the corpse reviver.
Signs and Symptoms: food poisoning which renders the patient prostrate (see *Arsenicum*); debilitating acute illness; severe exposure; after being almost drowned; patient lies apparently dead to the world with no reactions; extremely weak; flatulent; wanting fresh air; wanting the air conditioner on, whilst blue, very cold and collapsed.

CHAMOMILLA Teething

This remedy is mainly for children who are teething, though it is not a panacea, and there are other remedies for this. A keynote indication that the child needs *Chamomilla* is when you feel driven to distraction by their state. The child commonly complains a great deal, and is impossible to please.
Note: All cases of teething may include fever, irritability and sleeplessness.
Signs and Symptoms: teething; earache; tummy ache; problems caused by anger; mad with pain; one cheek hot, the other pale and cold; wants to be and is better being carried; moaning; earache; swelling; heat driving the infant frantic; worse at night; sweating; grass-green stools that may smell of bad eggs.

Other remedies for teething include the following:

KREOSOTUM

Signs and Symptoms: teething with restlessness; cross; willful; obstinate; rapid decay of teeth.

KALI BROMATUM

Signs and Symptoms: teething with fear and anxiety at night; night terrors with squinting, recognises no one.

APIS

Signs and Symptoms: teething with red, shiny gums; swollen like bee sting; shrieking.

TEREBINTHINA

Signs and Symptoms: teething with flying into temper; glossy tongue; enormous tummy; green stools; worms.

RHEUM

Signs and Symptoms: teething with very strong, sour smell; shrieking.

PHYTOLACCA

Signs and Symptoms: teething with biting hard on something to relieve pain; must bite teeth together; slow teething; weeping.

MERCURIUS, NATRUM MUR, SILICEA

Signs and Symptoms: teething with excess saliva.

CINA

Signs and Symptoms: very irritable; grinding teeth; screaming; cross; ugly; wants rocking; pain so sudden it shocks; stiffens with pain; worse being looked at; variable appetite; touchy in extreme; wants to be carried to no benefit; caresses have no effect; hitting, throwing things; a general exaggeration of the behaviour of Chamomilla children.

COCA *(COCA PLANT)* **Height Sickness**

Coca leaves are chewed by the indigenous peoples of the Andes mountains. It produces exceptional vigour and great endurance, even with poor nourishment and lack of sleep. People are able to travel great distances on foot up the mountains, and sustain themselves at high altitudes, by taking Coca. The 'mountain' can be psychological, spiritual or physical, because under the influence of Coca, people reach higher planes of existence, experience beautiful visions and gain an awareness of the sublime. Hence its use, and because it is addictive, abuse by some.

Signs and Symptoms: mountain/hot air ballooning sickness; dizziness; difficult breathing; exhaustion.

Note: If Coca fails to work, use *Arsenicum*.

COCCULUS *(INDIAN COCKLE)* **Travel Sickness**

Signs and Symptoms: travel sickness from cars, boats etc.; loss of sleep from night nursing, night shifts, etc.; giddiness from lack of sleep and travelling; nausea merely looking at food. This remedy is good for sensitive, introspective, kind children and adults.

Other remedies for car sickness include the following:

PETROLEUM

Signs and Symptoms: must stoop with the sick feeling, as if drunk; fears death is near; pain in back of head.

SEPIA

Signs and Symptoms: aversion to family; irritable; easily offended; best left alone; sudden weak feelings; heaviness; empty feeling not helped by eating; giddy; darkness in vision.

Other remedies for seasickness include the following:

NUX VOMICA
Signs and Symptoms: giddiness and moments of unconsciousness; hangover feeling, great irritability; nausea and vomiting; bitter taste; hiccups; wanting to vomit, but not being able to; over-sensitive to everything; faintness.

TABACUM
Signs and Symptoms: unpleasant, faint sinking feeling in pit of stomach; giddiness on getting up or looking up; better on deck in cold fresh air, and after vomiting; anxiety.

STAPHISAGRIA
Signs and Symptoms: easily offended; hiding anger and smiling sweetly.

Treatment: Try taking the remedy before and during travelling, every half hour if severe, or every time you feel bad again. Switch to another remedy if after a few attempts one does not work.

COLOCYNTHIS (BITTER CUCUMBER) Severe Pains, Colic
The symptoms that can be treated by *Colocynthis* are often caused by anger and frustration. When treating a fractious infant for colic with this remedy, it is best to treat the parents too, as the child may be ill in response to inner problems they can not yet voice.
Signs and Symptoms: nerve pains such as sciatica, neuralgia (head/face pain); pain in the ovaries; colic; feeling of being caught in a vice; sudden violent, cramping, radiating, cutting, grinding, griping, pinching, boring, gnawing, tearing pains which make the patient twist, scream and

double up; pains better from hard pressure like doubling up; heat; pain in waves; before dysentery-like stools.

Note: From eating something very bitter such symptoms may be expected, which clearly demonstrates the homeopathic principles of provings and like curing like.

CHINA (PERUVIAN BARK) Pick-Me-Up

Quinine is extracted from Peruvian Bark, and *China* is very useful in people supposedly cured of malaria yet with long-lasting low energy, or where one parent had malaria.

Signs and Symptoms: pick-me-up after excessive loss of blood, food poisoning (see above); after loss of other body fluids, such as diarrhoea (especially from eating spoiled fish), and long-lasting discharges and suppurations (long-lasting pus); after childbirth, where there has been excessive loss of blood; malaria; exhausted; weak; over-sensitive, especially to noise, light and pain; apathetic.

CRATAEGUS (HAWTHORN BERRIES) Weak Hearts

This remedy is a great heart tonic for the aged. It is said to act as a solvent on deposits in the arteries and heart — without side-effects — and in general to improve the action of the heart.

Treatment: Five drops in a wine glass of water three times a day for a number of months in order to get a long-lasting effect.

GELSEMIUM (YELLOW JASMINE) Influenza, Panic Attacks

In chronic illness, *Gelsemium* is for people who panic and need the loo.

Signs and Symptoms: influenza; panic attacks; feeling of great heaviness; eyelids feel like they need match sticks to hold them open; fever and chills which follow each other; virtually no thirst; tremendous drowsiness. (If you have flu and are too drowsy even to look up which remedy to use, then *Gelsemium* is probably what you need. So remember this one fact about flu!); better from profuse urination; slow onset of complaints.

Other flu remedies include the following:

BRYONIA
(see above)

EUPATORIUM PERFOLIATUM
Signs and Symptoms: violent, aching pains; great restlessness from the pains, yet wants to be still.

BAPTISIA
Signs and Symptoms: sore, heavy and aching muscles, with rapid prostration; the bed feels too hard, yet you are too weak to move; putrid odours; body feels like it is in pieces; appears drunk, drowsy, stupid and languid.

NUX VOMICA
Signs and Symptoms: irritable; chilled; can't bear to be uncovered; worse for motion.

PYROGEN
Signs and Symptoms: aching bruised soreness; very offensive discharges; sweating does not reduce fever; chill felt in bones; quickly oscillating temperature; pulse goes in opposition to fever.

ARNICA

Signs and Symptoms: sore and aching all over. (See First Aid, pages 24–6.)

Other remedies for panic attacks include the following:

ACONITE

Signs and Symptoms: instant expectation of death.

ARGENTUM NIT

For people who are great anticipators, impulsively rushing against imaginary deadlines.

OPIUM

Signs and Symptoms: sleepiness.

STRAMONIUM

(see below)

IGNATIA (ST IGNATIUS BEAN) Grief, Disappointed Love and Loss

Ignatia is the main remedy for acute grief, especially to help in preventing an older person who has lost their spouse from dying of grief for the other person. *Ignatia* oils the wheels of the grieving mechanism, and gets the tears flowing.

Signs and Symptoms: acute grief after the death of someone close; disappointment in love (especially for young person whose first love has not worked out); responds badly to consolation; believes it is best not to talk about it; broods silently; becomes sick; sighing incessantly; doesn't want to eat fruit.

Other remedies for grief include the following:

NATRUM MUR
Signs and Symptoms: very closed; can't cry; hates consolation; wants to be left alone; prefers salt.

CAUSTICUM
Signs and Symptoms: after death of a child, and where there have been several serious episodes of grief in the past which may be leading to partial or complete paralysis (lost voice, incontinence or multiple sclerosis).

PHOS AC, OPIUM
Signs and Symptoms: grief and drowsiness.

GELSEMIUM
(see above)

MEDORRHINUM (GONORRHOEAL VIRUS) After Effects of Gonorrhoea or NSU

This is a deep-acting remedy made from gonorrhoea. Anyone who has had gonorrhoea or NSU (non-specific inflammation of the urethra) will know about its effects. If the symptoms spontaneously recur after initial treatment with antibiotics, a patient will most likely need this remedy. Otherwise he or she will inevitably become sicker over time. This very common phenomenon needs thorough eradication by use of this remedy, but only through prescription by a professional homeopath.

THUJA, NITRIC ACID
Signs and Symptoms: when a person has acquired warts from sexual contact with another, even if they were burnt

off by laser or other treatment.

Note: Once the warts have taken root they are in the system and will slowly create damage. These warts require skilled, professional help.

LACHESIS, LYCOPODIUM, MERCURY Sore Throats

Sore throats can be acutes, but are often the result of a chronic inner problem. There are numerous distinct characteristics to sore throats; some of these are listed below, with the appropriate remedy indicated. All sore throats are sore and red.

LYCOPODIUM

Signs and Symptoms: sore throats go from right to left, or stay on the right; worse after sleep and from cold drinks.

LACHESIS

Signs and Symptoms: sore throats go from left to right, or start or stay on the left; worse from swallowing and hot drinks; throat very sensitive to touch; pain extends to the ear; they feel behind or above themselves.

LAC CANNINUM

Signs and Symptoms: sore throats oscillate from one side to the other frequently; they feel behind or above themselves.

MERCURY

Signs and Symptoms: increased saliva which patient may swallow; metallic taste; pain extends to the ear on swallowing; worse at night.

Other remedies for sore throats include the following:

ACONITE

BELLADONNA

NUX VOMICA **Hangover**
Signs and Symptoms: hangover.

PHYTOLACCA *(POKE ROOT)* **Breast Inflammation (Mastitis)**
This remedy for mastitis (in humans and animals) was convincingly demonstrated on BBC television. Half a herd of eighty cows was given *Phytolacca* — a few drops monthly in the drinking trough — the other half antibiotics, when sick with mastitis. The incidence of mastitis differed from nineteen to one (and this one was due to injury) over six months.
Signs and Symptoms: mastitis; inflamed nipples.

Other remedies for mastitis and inflamed breasts include the following:

BELLADONNA
Signs and Symptoms: red, hot and burning; very sensitive to touch.

BRYONIA
Signs and Symptoms: too painful to move at all; inflamed nipples.

SILICEA, LAC CANNINUM, PULSATILLA
Signs and Symptoms: pain while nursing.

URTICA URENS

Signs and Symptoms: insufficient or excessive breast milk.

Note: Consult a professional for these problems, but try
Urtica urens as a first step. (See page 28.)

STRAMONIUM (THORN APPLE) Birth Trauma

This is a remedy especially for birth trauma where the
baby is delayed at the second stage of delivery. There may
be suffocation, and the baby will be very frightened of
dying. They lie in terror of dying, panicking, and then they
are born. If such a baby is not immediately bonded with
the mother, then such terror will remain. He or she may
later wake up with night terrors, or as an adolescent or
adult be scared to go out and also to be alone —
especially at night — or even become schizophrenic.
Therefore separations after any birth should be avoided
whenever possible; if there is an unavoidable separation,
seek professional homeopathic help as soon as possible. It is
also even more important to breast feed in these
circumstances.

Signs and Symptoms: birth trauma; terror of dying,
panicking prior to birth; dreams of wet hairy places, a light
at the end of the tunnel and about Noah's Ark; desire for
light; fear of water, drowning, suffocation, tunnels;
claustrophobic; deep sense of isolation; abandonment.

Remedies for night terrors include *Kali bromatum* and *Calc
carb*.

SULPHUR Skin Eruptions

Skin eruptions are chronic complaints in the main, and if
suppressed lead to asthma, attention disorder (ATD) and
even convulsions — all of which should be treated

professionally. The drug cortisone, commonly prescribed by GPs, should be avoided, as it may lead to even worse problems in the future. Do not self-prescribe sulphur — see a professional homeopath.

THUJA (ARBOR VITAE)

This remedy benefits many older people who had the smallpox vaccination.

Signs and Symptoms: antidote to the effects of smallpox vaccination; warts (which may have been removed, leaving long-lasting white spots); secretive; desire; aggravated by or hate onions.

THE TREATMENT OF ACUTE ILLNESS

> In assessing acute cases, you are not looking for a diagnosis or the common symptoms of illness, but rather how the person is responding to the illness.

It is important to look beyond the symptoms to how the patient is reacting. Acute case taking is relatively easy. You need to pay attention to the obvious, and to be precise. High fever is high fever, but measure it to be sure. 40°C (104°F) is high, but 39°C is not.

Ask the patient exactly what is wrong; get him to describe it *in detail*, then consider what is unusual in this situation. Often a patient is not articulate, so you also need to observe him carefully and take account of any idiosyncrasies. Discuss his attitude to thirst, food, movement, wants, aversions, play — what is different from normal?

What about sweating, odour, heat, cold, light, dark, lying, sitting, restless, still, position lying, discharges, urine

smell (easy with nappies), stools? Make a list of the
obvious. Believe what you see, hear, smell, feel. Trust your
gut instincts, especially when you normally find them
reliable.

Support from your doctor

If you are worried, visit your doctor and find out what is
wrong. Be quietly assertive; when given complex medical
words and diagnoses, don't be afraid to ask what they
mean. The doctor may mention possible serious
consequences, but ask about the *likely* consequences of the
illness. Don't be panicked into accepting prescriptions for
antibiotics, antipyretics, etc. These are a last resort — often
life saving, but not a cure.

Can you manage it?

If you are anxious by nature, particularly about a child,
either buy a good self-help family medicine book and
educate yourself to allay your fears, or stop self-prescribing
and visit a professional homeopath.

Getting support

If you feel you need support, consult a local homeopath
about yourself or your child; get 'on their books' so you
can then telephone for urgent advice and support while
you find your feet. Some homeopaths also have an acute
drop-in clinic.

Find out from your local homeopath about beginner's
classes for first aid and treating acute illnesses. There will
always be something that you need to discuss that no book
can easily answer, and classes are a more effective way to
learn — and more fun too.

OBTAINING REMEDIES AND PRESCRIBING

Most chemists supply homeopathic remedies, and they are all of an acceptably high standard. Homeopathic pills in shops and chemists are normally 6c potency, which is fine for most conditions. You can buy LMI — my preferred method — as an alternative from specialist homeopathic chemists, but there is not much difference between them.

Use the pills one at a time, ignoring instructions on the bottles. For acutes, I prefer to use one tablet in a glass of water, crushed, dissolved and stirred; one sip is then one dose. (I use LM1 the same way — see page 63 for further information.)

With acute illnesses such as headache, sore throat, earache, fever, hay fever, repeat the dose as needed, which may be every five minutes for a very high fever, or perhaps three times a day for hay fever. The basic rule is as soon as symptoms start returning, repeat.

In acute cases I expect easily identifiable, sure signs of cure. These include:

- going to sleep soon after taking the remedy, and waking up after quite a while saying 'I feel better'
- relief of symptoms for a while followed by return (repeat)
- feeling better in himself, with the suffering more localised; in effect: 'I'm OK, but my body is suffering', whereas before 'I'm suffering' was the refrain
- milder symptoms that are tolerable, given that the person has an infectious disease.

Note: Absence of appetite but continued thirst is a good sign in illness. Don't feed an acute illness, but do encourage the patient to drink.

If the remedy you chose doesn't work within a reasonable time — half an hour in an acute, depending on its intensity — you need to consider your prescription again. Take the following steps:

- repeat the same remedy if you are sure it is right
- change the remedy if you think you should, as soon as you think this is the right thing to do
- don't panic — get other help instead, or wait.

Useful tips to bear in mind are:

- in acute illnesses symptom pictures can change rapidly, and so may the remedy
- repeat a working remedy for a few doses after the cure to prevent relapses
- in acutes do not treat at the start; a fever is a good thing for example, and only needs help if something is not going well
- the longer you wait the surer the symptom picture and the more certain the remedy; it is easy to get the remedy wrong if you prescribe too quickly; in children's diseases the acute fever stage is proper functioning; only prescribe if it fails to progress, or the fever is too strong; if a child has measles, chicken pox, mumps or rubella and the rash fails to show, *Sulphur* will push it out; if the disease shows signs of complications, affecting the sex organs, eyes, etc., *Pulsatilla* will usually sort it out
- keep records of what you do.

EMOTIONAL TRAUMA

An emotional trauma such as a bereavement, rape, shock, great fear, violent attack or imprisonment can create severe inner reactions, which the affected person can be helped to process with the aid of homeopathy. Often people get stuck part way through a trauma recovery, at the point where it resonates deeply with a previous early life trauma or parental conditioning.

These 'stuck-in-trauma' states vary according to the nature of the trauma and the individual involved. The person may have an acute new state, or it may appear as an aggravation of the original constitution, according to her vitality. The latter needs the constitutional remedy, or a related one.

A person recovering from rape, for example, will most likely encounter denial, fear, terror and anger during recovery, whereas a person recovering from a bereavement will focus more on loss and grieving. A diagnosis like AIDS or cancer can create an emotional trauma, and denial is often the first stage of this.

Main Remedies for Trauma

Aconite
Sudden shock such as an unexpected death or crash.

Natrum mur
Denial; bottled up tears; indicated by eating more salty things.

Ignatia
Grief, bereavement and loss; bottled up tears with sighing.

Staphisagria
Rage; rape anger; effects of surgical procedures for women, such as episiotomies.

STRAMONIUM

Terror after attacks; bombs, etc.

It should be emphasised that the constitutional remedy is often required, which requires professional help.

My book *Emotional Healing with Homeopathy* (see 'Recommended Reading', page 119) focuses on these problems in detail.

CHAPTER FIVE

Consulting a Homeopath

This chapter concentrates on what happens during a consultation with a homeopath. I will take you through how I approach an interview with a patient.

TAKING THE CASE

Taking the case is finding out what is 'wrong' with the patient, and is the basis of prescribing. Great importance is placed upon it, and sufficient time — an hour at least — must be given to it. The keys to good case taking are listening, observation, clarification and objectivity.

At first, the patient has a story to relate, and at this stage the homeopath listens a lot and speaks very little to allow the patient to speak freely. This is important in many ways, but especially so as not to prejudice the sort of information the patient presents: the patient must set the agenda on a visit, not the homeopath. The homeopath will speak for the purpose of establishing a co-operative atmosphere, in which there is trust and confidentiality, enabling the patient to feel free to discuss her deepest problems. With some patients it is not difficult to get the necessary information, as they talk readily and extensively about their physical and emotional issues and difficulties. With more closed and shy people, however, it is necessary to establish a rapport and to start the interview with an open question like 'what brought you here?', and to allow them gradually to open up.

The homeopath seeks to record what the patient says in her own words. Homeopathy is based on patients' language, in which there are often vital clues. With patients who are very closed, more skill is needed to elicit information, but in fact the observation 'closed' already narrows down the remedy possibilities. While the patient is narrating her story, the homeopath keeps all his senses alert, writing down not only what he hears as closely as possible to the patient's actual words, but also what he observes and senses from the patient.

The homeopath may deduce from his observations and the patient's story that she is open, closed or animated; that the story is told in a dull monotone or hasty speech; in an embarrassed, shy, stuttering way; that it is seductive, weird, unreal, concrete, in great detail, vague, etc. He will observe the patient's posture. Is she sitting relaxed in the chair, or sitting on the edge, leaning forward with eagerness, or sunk back? Are her legs, arms, head, hands and feet still, or are they constantly moving and twitching? Does she smile a lot or never, laugh appropriately or inappropriately? Is she clean, super-clean or a bit dirty, untidy or scruffy? Homeopaths note their observations about texture, appearance, cleanliness, unusual marks, growths, swellings — there are hundreds of potentially useful observations to make.

The homeopath has to remain objective whilst also being genuinely empathetic, friendly and interested. He may want to feel great sympathy for a tragic story, terrible suffering, or indignation at an obvious injustice, which is difficult to resist. Responding and getting drawn in damages the homeopathic process, as it can distort the true picture of the mind-body characteristics of the patient and therefore prevent the homeopath from finding the correct remedy. Being objective and non-judgmental are essential qualities for every homeopath; these qualities constitute the image of the unprejudiced observer, something that

Hahnemann wrote extensively about, and which every
homeopath strives to achieve through training.

I listen until the patient dries up. Then I repeat a
question — perhaps 'anything else?' — or leave a definite
pause, and then usually more comes out. Very often the
patient says 'that's all', yet within seconds out comes more,
and later more and more. It's a near certainty that 'that's
all' means 'wait, more is to come'. Sometimes in response
to a question a patient says 'I don't know', but after a short
pause she has the answer.

A patient has first to empty her mind of what she
came with to the homeopath — what I call 'what she
thinks is wrong with her'. Then after another pause for
reflection, more inner thoughts can float in from her soul
and reflect off her now empty mind, as there is space for
them to be received. The patient then speaks and pauses
again; then there is a empty space in the mind; she pauses
again; then she speaks her thoughts again, perhaps a
number of times. I call this common process 'what is really
wrong'. Since the last information is probably the most
deeply hidden to the patient herself, it is often her central
problem, and can therefore act as the core of the case.

If the homeopath is not sufficiently aware, he will cut
the patient short. I have a device to ensure long
comfortable waits, however. I work at my computer,
looking up symptoms and analysing the case; the patient,
sitting patiently while I am busy, ruminates further and out
come even deeper, long-lost thoughts, which I add to my
information.

Once I have listened to the patient's story — typically
half an hour long — I need to fill in the bits she may
have missed, sometimes prising out half-forgotten
memories, or ask her for more background. I am especially

interested in finding the peculiar features of the person, and her reactions to disease or illness that are not explained by the pathology or any external circumstances — which in reality are mostly of her own creation too. One useful way of getting this important information is to ask the patient to give actual, detailed examples of what they are talking about (eliminating the intellectualising common in well-educated people).

Another way is when we reach the point when the patient says 'I don't know' in response to a question like 'why do you think that?' I know then I have reached a core piece of reliable information. For example, if a person says 'I'm scared of dogs', I might ask 'why?' She replies 'well actually I am scared of most things'. I ask 'do you know why?' Her answer is 'because I feel threatened by everything'. Again I ask why, and the answer is 'I don't know — I've always felt like that'. This is core information.

Therefore, when the story is complete in the patient's terms, I attempt to fill in the gaps (this is not always necessary). With good observation, the inner story that acts to create all the symptoms is largely visible. However, because of miasms based on past diseases, I try to complete her life story, by finding out about the personal and family history of disease, illness and crisis.

It may not be possible to collect accurately all the required information in the first consultation, for the reasons above, and a second interview may be needed. Often the homoeopath will need time to reflect and free himself from the story to become sufficiently objective, or just quietly to reflect on the case. However, with experience, good training and good observational powers, finding a remedy is possible at the time of the interview —

and sometimes even within a minute or so of the
consultation starting.

THE CASE ANALYSIS

In analysing a case the homeopath looks for what is
characteristic of the person's response to the disease, not
the disease itself. So if his ulcer is burning but relieved by
hot drinks, I consider the uncommon bit — relieved by
hot drinks — as this cannot be explained by pathology
and is unique to the patient. I also try to find clues to the
individual's response to living (really the same thing). I
then join them together in a coherent fashion to form a
connecting thread, or better still a hub with radiating
spokes — peculiar responses — which all clearly emanate
from this one basic inner process. Homeopaths call this
inner process a central delusion — for example, 'feeling
threatened' — as it cannot be explained rationally. It is
important to bear in mind that everyone is unique —
there are no two people on the planet the same, not even
identical twins, although there are a lot of common core
delusions in people.

Once I have the hub I am on fairly certain ground.
However, it may not be possible to get such clarity for
many reasons, such as the drugs the person is taking or has
taken in the past. For these situations I have other
strategies. For example, I may adequately identify the
spokes of the wheel without the hub, which add up to
one certain remedy, yet may not understand the hub. It is
in fact common to cure a patient with a remedy without
fully understanding them.

There are other, generally less accurate, ways of
prescribing when the facts are less obvious, but with
poorer results.

CLASSIFICATION OF THE SIGNS AND SYMPTOMS

In homeopathy, symptoms are identified according to how close they are to representing the core of the person, the generating hub of the disease. Therefore feeling and thought symptoms are high up in the hierarchy. I also consider how peculiar the symptoms are. For example, burning pains relieved by heat is unusual, as explained above, and so might be lying absolutely still in headache; even more so is a pulsation in the stomach during heat, or feeling suicidal at 1 a.m. These can add valuable spokes to the wheel.

By considering every symptom I can classify them as follows:

- *central delusion or feeling (the hub)*: feeling alone in the world, threatened, being a great person
- *thought or feeling*: guilt, hatred, sympathetic, lonely, strange, rare and peculiar: a personal reaction that cannot be explained by pathology
- *general*: that apply to the whole body — hot person, chilly person, restless, twitchy
- *to do with parts*: pain in a part, inflammation, abscess, asthma, paralysis, hay fever symptoms.

Most symptoms and signs are to do with parts, but are only the outcome of the central disturbance over the years.

REPERTORISATION: FINDING A SHORT-LIST OF POSSIBLE REMEDIES

The homeopathic repertory is an index of around 130,000 signs and symptoms of disease, usually held on computer or as a reference book, with a list of remedies associated with each sign or symptom. It forms the accumulated wisdom of homeopathy over the years.

The object of repertorising is to produce a short-list of possible remedies to be considered. The first step is to choose a set of rubrics — signs and symptoms — that best indicate the core issues of the person and the case as a whole. For example:

- scars that burn: *Arsenicum, Graphities, Hypericum, Ignatia, Lachesis*, etc.
- delusions of greatness: *Agaricus, Cannabis indica Graphities, Hyoscyamus, Ignatia, Lachesis, Platina, Syphilinum*, etc.
- pressure over a hard edge relieves: *China, Colocynthus, Ignatia, Lachesis, Nux vomica*, etc.

In this example, the two remedies with these characteristics are *Lachesis* and *Ignatia*.

CONFIRMING THE REMEDY CHOICE

Having decided the choice is between *Lachesis* and *Ignatia*, I can then go to the *Materia Medica* and compare the types of people likely to be Ignatia and Lachesis.

Lachesis types are verbose, talkative, vivacious and attacking.

Ignatia types are secretive, reserved, closed and careful about details.

These may seem poles apart, but in reality people merge a bit into one or another association with a remedy, without absolute distinctions. A little reflection by the homeopath generally results in a conclusion that a person is of one type rather than the other; this can be a subject for discussion with the patient. Homeopaths usually try to involve the patient in the process, as her education, co-operation and long-term concern for her own health are helpful towards the achievement of good results. It is also important to get away from the 'you patient, me God' image of doctoring of the past. The homeopath enters into a partnership, where the patient is in charge and is responsible for the help she seeks.

WHAT IF IT IS THE WRONG REMEDY?

When a homeopath gives the wrong remedy — where it is almost but not exactly right — it will usually be beneficial up to a point. It will not do any harm unless persisted in outside the common principles of homeopathic practice. It is very hard to cause harm with homeopathy, and stopping the remedy usually results in any harm evaporating. Certainly the great majority of incorrect prescriptions simply have no effect.

PROGNOSIS — HOW LONG WILL IT TAKE AND HOW MUCH CAN WE EXPECT?

It is unlikely that just one remedy will cure someone (though when it does this is very gratifying). During the analysis of the case I consider the longer-term disease influences — miasms — and what their probable impact will be. I formulate a treatment plan, with options according to how the patient responds. Generally I first try a deep-acting remedy, which may take a few prescriptions — depending on the person — and persist with it as long as it works (which may be months or years). But if there are strong miasms, and several of them, I will prescribe for these too if the first remedies do not deal with them.

Bringing about a deep and long-lasting cure is clearly a lengthy process, and it can sometimes be very difficult. The benefits can be felt by the patient for a very considerable length of time, however — perhaps for his or

her whole life. Homeopaths believe that the likelihood of
further disease is greatly reduced or even eliminated by a
course of successful homeopathic prescribing over a
number of years, resulting in a healthy and therefore
happier old age. Homeopaths hope that such a process will
in time become a normal activity for most people.

The exact prognosis for an individual case is hard to
make, but as a general rule, the less orthodox medication
the patient has had, the shorter the illness; the younger the
person, the quicker and easier will be the process of cure.
In long-standing cases of twenty or more years of
established pathology I do not expect dramatic changes,
although significant improvements are still possible.

PRESCRIPTION AND POTENCY

Classical homeopaths prescribe one remedy at a time in a
clearly understood procedure. They give the remedy and
watch the results. They are not easily convinced about
cure; they expect to see sustained curative action,
otherwise after a time they doubt the validity of a
prescription. So the basic approach is to prescribe, then
wait and see how the patient responds. (Some practitioners
prescribe every remedy they think is needed
simultaneously in complexes, or combinations; or in a
quick sequence. People with this approach are not true
homeopaths, as they violate virtually every principle and
practice of homeopathy in prescribing this way.)

Once curative action is established, the same remedy
may be used for years to good effect. In more difficult
cases a series of remedies will progressively improve the
patient's situation.

Potency is a vexed question in homeopathy. There are,
however, a few tried and tested approaches. I use LM1 or

6c in a glass of water for most acute and chronic cases. For daily use, put the pill or LM1 granule in a 100 ml bottle of distilled water, and bang the bottle hard ten times on an old book every day before use. Then put a teaspoonful into a glass of water, stir vigorously and take one sip as a daily dose, throwing the rest away and making a fresh glass each day.

This is a highly effective method of long-term, safe prescribing, provided you stop when the remedy acts towards cure or aggravation of symptoms and do not re-start until the curative action is exhausted (see Chapter Two, 'The History and Principles of Homeopathy').

The rule homeopaths follow is to prescribe either a low dose — 6c or LM1 — repeatedly until the remedy acts, then stop; or to prescribe one high potency dose. (In highly medicated cases such as asthmatics, other rules apply.)

WAITING AFTER PRESCRIPTION
If the patient gets better I wait. If she relapses for any reason I also wait. If she relapses for no reason after a reasonable curative process, I repeat the remedy with the same potency. Repeating the remedy too soon is a very common mistake. (In chronic serious pathology, other rules may apply.)

CURE
In chronic disease we expect deep changes.

On the inner level:
- change of situation of stress
- greater creativity

- softer and more adaptable if previously too hard, or stronger and more assertive if previously too yielding
- more expression of loving kindness and togetherness, less separation, hatred and aloneness
- fewer fears, phobias
- less anger, attack, guilt, anxieties
- more irritation as she wakes up to her situation
- more confidence
- an aggravation or worsening.

On the thought level:

- less dogmatic, fixed thoughts, more flexible, ability to listen more.

On the physical level:

- minor aggravation, or slight worsening for a while
- return of old symptoms in reverse chronological order is a good sign
- symptoms getting better inside and worse outside
- symptoms getting better higher up the body and moving down.

These are the general trends, but further explanation is needed. With a deep cure, the next level out from the core will aggravate, so feelings of anger or rage may surface in a person when an inner disturbance is resolved. Hatred may be a good sign that a cure of the central problem is taking place, but is not that common. Such a cure may be so profound that the person doesn't notice it, and only the comments of relatives, friends and astute observation can make her realise it has happened.

Marriages may break up when a docile patient suddenly feels stronger inside, and can therefore decide not to put up with violence or abuse any longer. In these situations it is desirable — but frequently not possible — to treat the other person before or as well.

Involving one member of the family (or the whole family) is often helpful in reporting the 'blind side' of the patient.

ANTIDOTING

Homeopathy is energy medicine, so anything that interferes with the energies of the body can be a good or bad influence on the homeopathic process. My experience is that the best approach to health creation is to do one thing at a time; it is then possible to be clear about the patient's response. This does not always work in practice, however, and the following factors can complicate homeopathic prescribing:

- medical drugs — especially cortisone and those for asthma
- recreational drugs such as cannabis, amphetamines and LSD
- other therapies like acupuncture (which is like a sister to homeopathy)
- chanting and some meditation practices done for a number of hours a day
- positive affirmations if they are glossing over the deep problem (which is common)
- coffee in large, strong doses, or taken regularly
- excessive alcohol
- strong herbs, aromas, oils etc. such as peppermint, camphor and menthol, as these have energising effects when used regularly.

People with severe problems may need strict regimes; psoriasis, for example, is usually aggravated by strong alcohol. Generally, homeopathy works better alongside a moderate lifestyle.

CHAPTER SIX

The Professional Homeopath at Work

THE SNAKE WHO COULDN'T STRIKE

his chapter will take you through an in-depth case history and analysis in order to illustrate how a homeopath works and thinks. It also shows the depth of influence a person's experience of life — including any trauma — can have on his or her well-being and vital force.

> The smallest details in a patient's life are important for the homeopath to create the whole picture that is necessary to find the appropriate remedy.

Note that the patient's words as spoken during the consultation are in quotes; my observations follow each quote.

LARISSA'S CASE

Larissa is a thirty-four-year-old surgeon. Ukrainian by birth, she now lives in another country; she is married, and six months pregnant. Larissa has brown hair, piercing blue eyes and an open face. Of medium build, she is 5 ft 6 ins tall, smiles a lot and has a pleasant disposition. I have her permission to write her story here — names and locations have been changed.

Larissa is suffering from a duodenal ulcer, frequent headaches and constant catarrh dropping down at the back of the throat. My observation and a question reveal that she has red moles on her body, over one hundred altogether.

THE CONSULTATION

'At fifteen years old I started smoking, and the pain in my
epigastrium appeared.' (She points to it with two fingers.)
This is a classic way of indicating an ulcer; in homeopathy
I call this rubric 'pain in small spots'.
'Seven months ago, a homeopath prescribed me *Lachesis*,
potency LM1, daily for two weeks.'

The original substance, a snake venom, was diluted one to
one hundred three times and one to fifty thousand once,
in liquid form in water, and banged repetitively and hard
between each dilution.

   This remedy was selected according to Larissa's
constitution — her state as a person, in mind and body.
She was very talkative, vivacious, open, extrovert and liked
singing. The pain was in small spots, with an empty feeling
in her stomach which no amount of eating would relieve,
and many other signs and symptoms to indicate a Lachesis
type. *Lachesis* is made from the venom of a South
American snake, and is a very popular homeopathic
medicine. All snake types (people) are venomous in speech,
striking to kill like venomous snakes (making a pain in a
small spot).

'Before taking the remedy I was depressed and anxious,
had strong fears about working nights in the hospital, and
strong headaches, and lots of personal problems. After
having *Lachesis* I became calm, my anxiety and sadness
disappeared, I slept and laughed a lot, and I was very much
better after it.

   'However, I then developed a severe pain in the area
of the ulcer, with nausea, and an extreme empty feeling
which nothing would fill, constant pain and spasm — very

intense and severe, then it would reduce — extending to shoulder and sternum. This was my old ulcer pain returning with a vengeance.'

This is a classic response in homeopathy: when a remedy works, old symptoms return briefly. However, because *Lachesis* was prescribed without sufficient patient education, and because Larissa was a doctor whose general approach to pain is to leap on it with pain killers, this reaction (the aggravation) was excessively severe. Larissa resorted to drugs to squash it, as the pain was too much to bear.

The prescription should have been to take the remedy daily until there was any noticeable reaction, then stop and wait. The reaction would then have been less dramatic, but perhaps even more effective. It is often best to use simple conventional drugs to manage pain, as they will probably only alleviate it, and not destroy the curative process.

My question was: she is clearly better so what else is there to do? It is very common that once a homeopathic remedy has worked its magic for the patient to ask 'can I have some more magic please?' This is not done directly, but by the patient simply forgetting what has been cured and focusing on what is left — things that previously she had relegated as unimportant. Homeopaths have to be on guard against this ploy, as new prescriptions can sometimes stop the initial good work in its tracks. The patient needs to be patient, and wait.

Over time there will often be a relapse into the old state.

There are two types of relapses: those with obvious causes, such as an overdose of alcohol, an emotional upset, a long flight; and those that occur slowly for no obvious reason. The relapses with causes will mostly pass with a natural recovery back to the improved state; as a rule of thumb I can say on the first relapse wait, because it will pass. When a slow relapse is happening, one without reason, a repeat prescription (more of the same remedy) will be required.

Sometimes it is important to prescribe quickly on the first sign of relapse — as in cases with serious pathology — because these people have a real battle to stay healthy and any relapse can herald a difficult recovery, if there is to be one at all. However for a relatively 'walking well' patient such as Larissa, the repeats should be minimised and this will result in the *shortest* cure, whilst unwise repeats or changing the remedy will lengthen the curative process: for the shortest route to a cure, the patient needs the least medication.

So not only do homeopaths use micro-doses of medicines in the shortest possible sequences, but they also repeat the medicine at less frequent intervals, to get the maximum effect.

I then asked Larissa to tell me what else was wrong. 'I'm lazy and inconsistent — I get keenly interested in things, then give up.'

In homeopathic terms this is: undertakes many things — persists in nothing.

'Back in the Ukraine, I presented the image of a strong person by suppressing my emotions, but it was only an image. I lack confidence — I work with great accuracy as I don't want to make mistakes.'

This is a common strategy of a sensitive person who hates

criticism — she becomes the perfect surgeon to avoid any possibility of humiliation.

'Because of my laziness I can't learn from text books, they are so boring. I only learn from practice, I will not read text books.'

Homeopathically this is aversion to reading.

'When my mother was pregnant with me they *never wanted* me. But once I was born my mother and father loved me from first sight, and after this I have been consistently loved and cared for.
'As a student I trained in fencing and karate, but I was never able to hit my opponent — there is always a wall between me and striking anyone. I just can't do it. I can be very angry, but I cannot be violent. I will smash things in extreme, throw something, but I won't hit someone.'

As Larissa had been to a homeopath before and had begun to study homeopathy, she was aware of what homeopaths are interested in and so she listed a whole string of things without my asking.

'I love animals, especially cats, to an extreme. I am scared of cockroaches and I love snakes.'

Few people are keen on cockroaches, but rarely before in a consultation has someone volunteered a love of snakes.

'I have had several repeating dreams since childhood, which continued until three years ago.'

Repeating dreams tell about the unresolved driving forces within a person, and are the things that best indicate the inner, unconscious motivation.

'In my first dream I'm in a container which I can't get out of — however many legs I get over the side, I am still stuck.'

I inquired as to how many legs she had, but to no avail, I wonder if it's a spider or a centipede, or what is in the container?

'Another dream is of being persecuted. It's a very vivid dream, and I see everything like a movie. I am running, and it's a crime film.'

This dream might represent the person's ego in full flight from her soul, because the ego would be seen to be a delusion in the spotlight of the soul, a mere fabrication without substance. Lachesis people normally have strong feelings of persecution.

'In another dream I'm in a public place, about to perform or have to do something, but I can't, as there is something wrong with my clothes — they are torn or dirty. I am shy or anxious, and can't do it.
'The only dream that is current is a recurring one, in which I am going to live abroad.'

Larissa is in reality living abroad.

'But always there is an obstacle to my leaving — everyone else goes, but I am unable to, for example because my luggage is lost.'

Larissa then continued with general information.

'My mother controls everything in my life.
'Three months ago I developed a great fear of earthquakes, and thought every moment it will happen and the building, a block of flats I am in, will collapse and I will die, crushed under the building, or I neither live or die, but am stuck in pain. I am very scared of pain.
'Though I am lazy, I like to knit and make tapestry. I just can't relax while sitting, and must be active somehow with my fingers.'

While telling me all this she is playing with her fingers a lot.

'I sleep in the embryonic position on my right side, and I can't sleep on my left.'

In homeopathy some remedy types are known to have preferences for sleeping on the front (Medorrhinum, Pulsatilla), the right side (Phosphorus, etc.), the left side, back, can't sleep on back because of nightmares etc. Phosphorus, Lachesis and Arsenicum people sleep on the right and can't sleep on the left. Pulsatilla and Mercurius people, amongst others, sleep in embyonic positions.

'I like to make public presentations and to be in public, and I sing in a chorus, but I can't sing solo except under the influence of alcohol. I am very chilly, and can't bear heat or cold.'

The aversion to heat is strange for such a chilly person. I call such people thermometers, as they are so sensitive to temperature.

'When I lived in the Ukraine I didn't allow myself to cry, but since living here I cry within the family and have become softer, and I am not so critical, but strangely more often ill.

'At the age of twenty-one or two, I had a strong allergy to wild strawberries, and came out in large hives, red and swollen over my whole body up to my head, for which I used antihistamines, etc. I have some remaining spotty effects on my face. I also have constant post nasal discharge.'

ANALYSING THE CASE

There are immutable principles involved in holistic-homeopathic case analysis, as described earlier in the book. At the same time, however, there are many different practical ways of approaching an individual case, each one seeking to come to a core understanding of the patient. One such approach is to try to understand the different aspects of the case as pieces of a jigsaw, and then to put the pieces together and see if it makes a recognisable picture.

SIGNIFICANT FEATURES OF THE CASE

Larissa:

• *can't* hit or strike opponents in martial arts
• *can't* get out of the pot
• *can't* fill the empty feeling however much she eats
• *can't* make a journey
• *can't* go solo in public
• *can't* persevere, gives up easily
• *can't* learn from text books
• *can't* control her own life.

It seems that whatever she wants to do in life, her path is blocked by a 'can't do', and I conclude that she is obstructing herself because of some internal edict called 'can't do'. Another way of thinking about this is to see it as a central delusion, an unconscious process that she cannot explain and is unaware of the reason for, that explains her whole mode of living. A core delusion is the 'mother' of all her smaller delusions.

A second peculiar aspect is this: she is an abdominal surgeon, and yet she has a fear of pain. In my little experience of surgery and surgeons, it is all to do with performing painful operations, and avoiding pain in the process. It seems significant to me that Larissa specialises in inflicting pain, yet at the same time has a specific fear of pain.

At this point I am gathering together all the information without any general plan, allowing the jigsaw pieces of a life to form — hoping that at some point I can see enough of the pieces and bring them together to see the whole picture.

I am struck by the timing of her pregnancy. She is now six months pregnant, therefore she became pregnant one month after the prescribing of *Lachesis*. I ask why she decided to get pregnant when she did. She says that she had a family discussion with her husband and her mother, and together they agreed it was time. This confirms her comment that her mother controls her life.

Yet I wonder if this is truly what happened. My guess is that at thirty-four years old and happily married for some years, this discussion had taken place many times before to no avail. My guess is that after the *Lachesis* she was much more connected to her inner being, and her natural maternal feelings have arisen (or descended). As a consequence of taking the remedy, the whole family 'psychological network' has changed. Lachesis people

usually have a strong egotism, and I would have expected
this to soften.

To me, the pregnancy strongly supports the idea that
the remedy is working, as does the fact that she is now
studying homeopathy. I believe it is because she was
astounded by the effect of the *Lachesis*.

LARISSA'S ORIGINAL TRAUMA

Another interesting aspect of the case is her fear of
earthquakes. Why, three months into her pregnancy, does
this occur for no apparent reason, when she did not have
this fear before? What happens at three months in a
pregnancy? Of course — when she was three months old
in her mother's womb, we know she was unwanted, so in
all probability her mother was thinking of aborting her.
Picture the scene. Her mother was thinking: 'Shall I kill
her? It's so difficult — I will have the responsibility. It will
dramatically affect my life — the restrictions, the money,
the support ... But I can't kill her — it's against my nature,
it's murder, I can't do it.' This dilemma raged inside the
mother for weeks, maybe even as an on-going discussion
with her husband. (At this point in the analysis, I asked
Larissa about the abortion idea, and she confirmed that her
mother told her this).

So now she has a three-month-old foetus inside her,
and relives her own experience of threatened life and
death, in the womb, as earthquakes, the building
collapsing, life and death. This puts the next piece of the
jigsaw in position, and the whole picture is starting to fall
into place.

Why the 'can't do' pattern of her life, however? This is
because her mother, at the point of abortion, could not kill
her, as her love of life prevailed. So Larissa is stuck at the

life and death point of her original trauma — can't hit, can't journey on, 'can't do'. You can picture her mother screaming to herself 'I can't do it'. The next piece of the jigsaw is now in place.

For what other reasons do I know that the trauma took place in the womb and not after her birth? The answer lies in the fact that she sleeps in the embryonic position — the last place where she felt safe, just before three months' gestation were over following her conception. The 'can't do' theme is so all-embracing because the trauma took place before the baby's senses and feelings developed; it is profoundly in the unconscious mind. In fact, it is primitive.

Why is she an abdominal surgeon? This is the skill you need to carry out an abortion, or to create life for a stuck child — which she feels she is — by performing a caesarian delivery. She is a 'stuck embryo'. This may seem far-fetched, but I have seen this sort of correlation countless times.

Larissa is successful in spite of the 'can't do' aspect of her life because the trauma is buried by a lot of love from the time of her birth. It is profoundly unconscious. All her memories tell her that her parents always loved her.

WHY IS LARISSA STILL CONTROLLED BY HER MOTHER?

Her mother had control of her life during the critical decision of whether to have an abortion — only by her mother's grace was she allowed to live. It is therefore hardly surprising, given that she is stuck at this place emotionally, that even now she feels under her mother's control. She 'can't do', and her mother has control of her life (and death).

THE NEXT STAGE

Now that I understand the formative trauma, the central
state or delusion, what can I do about it? Larissa may be a
Lachesis type — Lachesis is a poisonous snake that under
attack strikes out to kill, yet she cannot do this. There are
hundreds of non-poisonous snakes that cannot kill. Is she
one of the ones we don't know about? I know that the
remedy *Lachesis* worked in the past to a highly significant
degree, and I can now look up in the homeopathic rubric
(signs and symptoms) index to see which remedies
correspond to the facts I have.

Signs and symptoms:

- dreams of being pursued
- dreams of unsuccessful efforts to do various things
- undertakes many things but does not persevere in
  them
- love for animals
- inconstancy
- dreams of journeys
- delusions she was about to die
- fear of pain
- plays with fingers
- restless fingers
- alcohol ameliorates
- singing
- ailments from stage-fright
- stomach emptiness not relieved by eating
- strawberries aggravate
- stomach pain sensation in a spot
- stomach ulcer
- stomach pain extending to sternum
- stomach pain extending to shoulders
- heat and cold aggravate

- sleeps on the right and can't sleep on the left
- aversion to reading.

While these are not all *Lachesis* signs and symptoms, the great majority are, so the picture essentially adds up to *Lachesis*. Parental roles have an important part to play in finalising the picture. At conception, the parents are the God and the Goddess; at birth, they are the King and Queen; they then become friends or 'brothers and sisters' around fourteen years.

Bearing this in mind, there are two rubrics that clearly confirm *Lachesis*:

- delusion under control of superior being (her mother, when a three-month-old foetus)
- undertakes many things, but perseveres with none of them ('can't do' idea).

Lachesis is the only remedy common to both.

REMEDY

I know that *Lachesis* has already worked as a remedy, because it brought about considerable changes in Larissa's feelings — a pregnancy, studying homeopathy, and a temporary worsening of her physical symptoms, all classical signs of cure in homeopathy. The explanation for her seeing me for more help is probably due to the incomplete action of the remedy, as it is possible it was cut short by the drugs she took to ease the aggravation of the returning ulcer pain. It is then easy to prescribe more of the same, but as I wish to prevent another aggravation, I recommend:

- first one dose LM1, by three-glass method
- if after one week there has been no effect, one dose by single glass method

- if after one further week there has been no
  effect, one dose a day for up to a week, stopping at
  the first sign of any effect.

This should minimise the aggravation, and allow a deeper
cure to take place. It is also less common for second doses
to aggravate.

OUTCOME

Larissa's fear of earthquakes disappeared, and she continued
to have a peaceful pregnancy. All that was needed was
more time for the original prescription to work.

Note: It is quite safe to treat a pregnant woman with
homeopathic remedies — in fact there can be highly
desirable reasons to do so. In cases where women have
experienced very frightening births themselves, treating
them for this while pregnant will increase the possibility of
their giving birth without fear.

CONCLUSION

The point I am elaborating through this case is not the
prescription but the analysis.

The core of every chronic case is what most people
die of — and this is happening in most long-term
disease in the western world today.

The pathology, the life style and the career closely reflect the primary emotional trauma. However, the primary emotional trauma may not be a single event, but may be of a variety in which there is a repeating process. For example, if a parent repeatedly threatens a young child every time she does something the parent does not want with 'if you do that again ... I'll hit you ... ' then the child grows up in fear, feeling threatened, and will live her life with these feelings.

If the homeopath can understand the formative forces in a person, then he or she has a better chance of selecting appropriate rubrics and remedies. It is also then possible to begin to comprehend the meaning of symptoms and disease.

For example: stomach, empty feeling, unrelieved by eating, can be seen as reflecting a life which is empty and unrelieved by the edict 'can't do'. Delusion under control of superior power equals mother when you are in the womb. I can imagine many cases with this symptom, coming from similar beginnings but with less loving parents.

In Larissa's case the central edict is something like 'to do is to die', and 'my life is under the control of a superior being'.

> At a deep level, all disease and symptoms are lower and higher delusions which come from the primary delusion. All pathology is based on illusions.

It might be that Larissa could be fully cured by *Lachesis*. Yet the hundred or so red moles and the excessive post-nasal catarrh point to an underlying miasm, the 'after effect' or the 'history of a disease' rather than the disease

itself. It is therefore likely that there will need to be a
second prescription at some time.

Lachesis should continue to do Larissa a lot of good.
Later on some new signs and symptoms will arise,
combine with left-over old rubrics, and together form a
new picture. By this time she will be a quantum leap
ahead in terms of health and happiness. But, given time,
she will complain about these new but lesser symptoms
almost as vigorously as the original ones. I will then have
to consider the options based on these new symptoms.

It is possible that other remedies may be needed; these
are likely to be *Nitric acid* and *Thuja* — but this is now the
time to wait and see.

CHAPTER SEVEN

Chronic Diseases

Chronic diseases often start slowly, or with a flourish, and once started continue along a never-ending path which restricts, maims and may finally kill the individual. Easily identifiable examples of these are alcoholism, heart disease and cancer.

Samuel Hahnemann identified the basic causes of chronic diseases in *Chronic Disease*, published in 1828 — many of his perceptions are still ahead of the times today.

Hahnemann believed (as we do now) that adverse influences on health include poor diet, alcohol and modes of living — cold, damp, unhygenic conditions, polluted water and air. Many of these conditions have been improved by better sanitation, better housing and primary health care. However, Hahnemann did not see them as primary causes of diseases — unless they are carried to great excess such as famine — but rather as secondary to deeper factors. Given twentieth-century advances, most of today's diseases in the western world come from internal processes within us.

Inherited diseases and trauma still predispose people towards unhealthy living — alcoholism, for example. In dealing with these predispositions it is important to educate the population about the effect of alcohol, because once established, addictions are hard to break.

Hahnemann particularly identified diseases that come from a few inherited or acquired illnesses and from emotional trauma.

THE EFFECT OF INHERITED AND ACQUIRED DISEASES

Hahnemann's pioneering observations on the nature of human suffering led him to some startling and profound conclusions. He began to develop this train of thought after observing that some of his most carefully selected remedies failed to achieve lasting results and that the patients relapsed. This led him to seek underlying pathological factors (research that lasted eleven years) which he referred to as the 'miasmatic state'.

> The miasmic state is the underlying susceptibility fundamentally responsible for the acute and chronic diseases from which people suffer.

In his work Hahnemann isolated three miasms:
- psora — the 'itch', 'the mother of chronic disease', an underlying weakness or susceptibility
- gonorrhoea
- syphilis.

These miasms can be inherited or passed on from generation to generation. Modern research shows that the DNA of certain viruses can be incorporated into the genetic material of cells and thus passed on to future generations — confirming the miasm concept. In-depth study of these miasms leads to the exploration of human suffering from its origins at the beginning of civilisation to their present manifestations as all the known diseases.

To paraphrase Hahnemann: incalculably greatest and most important is the chronic effect of the 'itch' infection which, after the internal infection of the whole organism, announces itself as present by a skin eruption. Sometimes this consists only of a few vesicles accompanied by intolerable, voluptuous itching (and a peculiar odour). *This monstrous internal chronic miasm is the only fundamental cause and producer of all the other innumerable forms of disease.* These diseases come under the following names: nervous debility, hysteria, hypochondriasis, mania, melancholia, imbecility, madness, epilepsy and convulsions of all sorts, softening and curving of the bones, caries, cancer, gout, piles, jaundice, dropsy, amenorrhoea, bleeding from the stomach, nose, lungs, bladder and womb, asthma and ulceration of the lungs, impotence, sterility, migraine, deafness, cataract, paralysis, defects of the senses and pains of thousands of kinds.

Hahnemann makes similar observations about the effect of the acquired diseases syphilis and gonorrhoea, both sexually transmitted. This was of course well before modern scientific advances measured the three stages of syphilis and identified its process of inner destruction from ulcer to severe nerve damage and other effects. Hahnemann saw, by close observation, that the syphilitic ulcer which occurs at the first site of infection after a period of inner gestation and the figwart (growth of tissue) that likewise occurs at the first site of gonorrhoeal infection, are the beginnings of two more tremendous diseases. Syphilis is now universally recognised as a pernicious, invasive disease with far-reaching consequences, which cannot be cured merely by suppressing the ulcer. Recent surveys in the UK show that twenty per cent of people with syphilis still have it after treatment.

Researchers such as Harris Coulter in his book on AIDS (acquired immune deficiency syndrome) even demonstrate that AIDS bears a close resemblance to third-

stage syphilis, and this may yet prove to be right. We now
know that from the instant of contagion it immediately
moves through the nerves and blood to invade the whole
organism; without systematic monitored eradication, it will
continue to develop over years and invade the whole
psychosomatic being, leading to slowly developing stages
of degradation.

Medical science has yet to accept that warts, moles
and skin tags are the third stage of the gonorrhoea
infection, and that cutting off or lazering warts does
nothing to stop the inner process manifested outwardly as
warts from spreading and creating chaos within. More
importantly, medical science has also yet to appreciate that
suppressing all forms of eruptions, ulcers, warts, itch,
eczema etc. is to suppress or ignore a very powerful disease
process in the making.

Suppression of the original itch disease only serves to
hide it away while it builds up within and develops into
one of the myriad shapes which form the thousands of
non-sexually transmitted diseases that afflict the human
race. Hahnemann asserts that all disease has its foundation
in the three miasmatic states.

PSORA — THE ITCH

Psora dates from pre-Christian times, to leprosy and 'St
Anthony's Fire'; these skin diseases may have come from
one primary disease now lost in history, but which is
basically the itch. For a long time leprosy was isolated, so it
may have been held in check. As it was suppressed, its
suppressed version was able to spread without limit.
Leprosy is not normally cured, but suppressed by treatment
over centuries. Homeopaths believe that it is passed on
genetically, as an inner process that does not manifest itself.

For thousands of years, all sorts of ointments were used to suppress the itch, but the best was Sulphur, which often cures it homeopathically (as in like cures like). It was found that mineral baths helped the itch, and Sulphur occurs at high levels in mineral waters. However, if it is not potentised, repeated doses of Sulphur will fail. Commonly the quantity was increased in the form of the application of Sulphur-based ointments, which suppressed the itch. If applied long enough, the ointment suppressed it for good, and only later would an apparently unrelated disease occur. Sulphur has been replaced by cortisone to suppress all forms of irritation, on the skin and in the lungs (asthma is the itch in the lungs). It is highly effective as a suppressant, and only very strong constitutions fail to respond to its effects.

The effects of suppressed or hidden, slumbering itch cover fifty pages in Hahnemann's *Chronic Diseases*. It is quite clear that communities throughout the world are affected — it is so contagious, and the opportunities for contagion are so numerous.

Hahnemann identified suppressed itch by careful, methodical observation and reading. The following are some of the diseases and conditions he identified as having their origin in suppressed itch:

worms in children; one-sided headaches; falling out and dry hair; sweaty head on going to sleep; easy sweating on least exertion; numbness from slight causes; swollen neck glands; paleness; eye inflammations; cracked tongue; cramps in the calves; frequent colds; frequent attacks of difficult breathing; easily chilled; continuous blockage of the nostrils; very cold hands or feet; smelly feet; heat flushes; easy spraining; hard stools; corns; period problems; empty feeling in stomach; piles; swollen veins; pains worse from rest; frequent boils; vivid dreams; unrefreshing sleep; extreme dislike of milk; chilblains; cracking in the joints; when every skin cut festers; dry skin; scaly spots on skin; itching vesicles that burn after rubbing.

None of these is a really serious illness — this is the state of the slumbering itch, the sort of thing that a quick trip to the doctor will fix. The problem is compounded once you suffer a severe trauma — such as a car accident, the loss of someone close, a difficult marriage — which results in an acute illness. When this acute illness is treated by modern drugs which react upon this slumbering giant, it then arises within you and takes hold. What started as frequent colds suppressed with antibiotics becomes sequentially bronchitis, then chronic asthma, or glue ear, allergies, etc. Likewise, eczema treated with cortisone becomes hyperactivity (an itchy brain) or asthma, convulsions or epilepsy.

Symptoms that arise will be further attacked by doctors unwittingly, without knowing their origin; within a few months, years or even a decade, much apparently unrelated disease will erupt, under the conscientious attention of a well-intentioned health care system using powerful drugs.

Hahnemann wrote that latent chronic disease in young people can be quickly eradicated, provided it is well managed (and this means not interfered with by prescriptions of antipyretics, antibiotics, anti-inflammatories, anti-histamines, etc.). In a person who has experienced from ten to twenty or thirty years of chronic disease, however, the process can take a year or so, and later it becomes incurable. The three primary disease influences make the process more complicated; and if severe traumas such as a bad birth experience, violence or sexual abuse especially are added to the addictions that often follow such histories, then cure becomes a work of great skill and patience.

To summarise, the itch is lack, reduction, poverty, absence, lowered vitality. Sycosis (what Hahnemann called the long-term effect of gonorrhoea) is excess, growth, over-production, etc.; the long-term effect of syphilis is destruction, depression and a physical and mental eating away of the person affected.

Hahnemann listed a few remedies to deal with the uncomplicated effects of the itch, gonorrhoea and syphilis:
• for syphilis, *Mercury*
• for the long-term effects of hidden gonorrhoea, *Thuja* or *Nitric acid*
• for uncomplicated itch, *Sulphur*.

A patient's requirements are usually much more complicated, however, and such curative ideas are only a starting point in treatment.

PSYCHOLOGICAL HEALTH

Hahnemann says that uninterrupted grief or frustration will multiply any small sufferings more certainly than all other bad influences. Today, we know that any severe emotional trauma that happened to you in the past — or to a parent — can affect your continuing state of health considerably. Dr Edward Whitmont, the leading homeopathic psychologist, says that many hard-driving types of attitude result in heart attacks, and that illnesses such as stomach ulcers and cancers frequently have emotional causes.

> Homeopaths see an intimate link between psychology
> and pathology — they are two expressions of the same
> thing.

Individuals can suffer deeply from inheriting emotional
traumas from a parent who lived with a buried, unresolved
rejection, war drama, or distant birth separation. These can
imbue the offspring with an emotional state of which you
have no memory at all.

It is often possible to see in families how the children
mirror their parents precisely. The personality traits they
have taken on from their parents include depressive
tendencies, fears, phobias, self-denial, self-criticism and lack
of confidence. Sound health-creating principles and
practices that work to interrupt and resolve this mirroring
over generations are essential.

GLOBAL HEALTH

A national consciousness, made up of affected individuals
and their families, can be affected too. For example, the
Japanese, having effectively denied their war experiences of
fifty years ago, have buried them deep inside their national
psyche. Only recently has there been any public
recognition of their humiliation, their war crimes in China
and use of captives as prostitutes and slaves; and there is
still a great resistance to opening up and acknowledging
the past. The effect has been to direct their energies into a
very effective economic 'war', in which they become a
dominant world power. Yet when this success begins to
fade, as the Pacific Rim countries and China take over,
where will those deeply buried inner traumas lead them?
The effect of the release of the suppressed feelings of those

in the former Yugoslavia is a prime example of what can happen.

These things can be seen in every country, including our own — old traumas overwhelming the natural loving state within each person. When groups of such people get together they can ignite a bushfire of hatred or revenge which may then engulf a whole country or area. The world state can be analysed and profoundly understood by applying the principles of modern physics, psychology and homeopathy.

> In essence, physics, psychology and homeopathy all say the same thing: health is not just a personal matter, but has profound global implications.

THE CHRONIC HEALTH PICTURE

Society has made great strides in hygiene and food production, and overcome poor physical living conditions in many parts of the world. And some progress has been made towards the stopping of wars (which leave severe emotional trauma in their wake, rippling on for centuries). But we are only beginning to wrestle with the problems of emotional trauma, abuse, war traumas, the effects of inherited disease such as gonorrhoea, the itch and syphilis. Modern conventional medicine, with its powerfully effective but suppressive drugs, is currently aggravating these problems, not helping them.

Pollution of all kinds is also on the increase. Food pollution is growing through poor farming practices — excess chemicals and cruel animal husbandry. Killing and eating well-kept animals is quite acceptable, in my opinion; it is eating cruelly kept animals, dosed with hormones and antibiotics, that carries with it high risk and potential damage in the human food chain. Male testicular cancer, for example, is reported to be linked to hormones routinely given to animals in their feed.

Free-living lifestyles, serial relationships and easy world-wide travel have multiplied the opportunities for sexually transmitted diseases. In addition, whereas a century ago there was high infant mortality, nowadays infant death is avoided by advances in medical care. Set against individual parents' joy at the survival of their young is the price — nature's device of rooting out the weak has gone. With two world wars this situation has been compounded by killing whole generations of our fittest men. My father was a sick man with a smouldering disease left over from earlier medical treatment; eventually the resulting complications killed him. He could not fight, and fathered four children, whereas my strong uncle died as a fighter pilot, without having had the opportunity to have children. In my case, I suffered twenty years of asthma.

Not only must we seek to keep newly born babies alive, but we must also seek to bring them rapidly to strong, vibrant health, otherwise we will breed a weaker race. Shepherds in Bulgaria used to be fit until they reached the age of one hundred years or so. Once they stopped living with the sheep up in the mountains, however, they began to die at eighty years of age. Their vigour was lost.

If the human race gets much weaker, then we will become more vulnerable to natural and man-made disasters in the form of a series of new deathly scourges like the plague or the effects of a nuclear installation getting out of control. The outbreak in the 1990s of the Ebola virus — a deadly and highly contagious disease —

in Mozambique, is a telling example. Had the outbreak not been contained, the effects could have been catastrophic on an international scale. To try to avoid this scenario, we need to make creating healthy people a national priority. Healthy means fit, happy, creative, kind, free of disease, and taking no conventional medicines. It also infers trauma–free birth experiences and better parenting. Health creation systems like homeopathy and education on healthy life styles, rather than disease maintenance systems like the conventional medicine of today, are vital to individual survival and to the survival and evolution of the human race.

CHAPTER EIGHT

Homeopathic Remedy Pictures

When taking a case, the homeopath builds up a picture of an individual which will fit one remedy more closely than any other — like cures like. There are numerous remedy families in homeopathy: gases; metals; minerals; radioactives; plants (whole plants, nuts, barks); animals (birds, fish, mammals, snakes, insects); and disease products (tuberculosis, syphilis). Within each of these there are sub-families with distinct qualities and characteristics.

> Nuts have hard outsides and remedies made from them suit people who are hard and tough. *Nux vomica* is for tough, ambitious business people, etc. (hard nuts!).

Poisons from creatures like tarantulas, black widow spiders, bees, wasps, hornets, scorpions, snakes, some fish, minerals like Arsenic and plants are used. The type of people for whom these form an appropriate basis for a remedy are those who make spiteful, poisonous remarks, are attacking, suspicious or jealous, etc.

There are analogous remedies on each plane of existence, yet each with its own characteristic expression and predisposition. For example, Hydrogen (gas) is appropriate for types who feel superior, as are Syphilinum (human disease), Eagle (bird), Cannabis Indica (plant), Granite (mineral), Platina (metal) and Plutonium (radioactive).

The following are examples of remedies from different sources, with an indication of the type of person for whom they are appropriate:

Gas: Hydrogen — for people with lofty intellectual ideas

Bird: Eagle — for those with an elevated or a detached view

Disease: AIDS — for those suffering severe abuse

Animal: Dog — for people with beaten up, adoring eyes

Insect: Tarantula — for those with spider-like activity

Mammal: Dolphin — for people with boundless love

Snake: Rattlesnake — for those who attack with warning, the rattle

Plant: Viola Odoratum — for people with a very intellectual form of superiority

Nut: Anacardium — for those who are hard cases

Mineral: Chalk (Calcarea Carbonicum) — for people who are soft, collapse easily

Metal: Gold — for those who shine the brightest

Radioactive: Plutonium — heaven and hell.

THE SNAKE FAMILY AS AN EXAMPLE

These are the characteristics of the snake family and their different uses. Every family of remedies has similar global characteristics as well as individual differences.

All snakes are jealous, suspicious, talkative, attracting, desire to strike, seductively magnetic, telling an advertising-like story about themselves, drawing you in, also feeling disadvantaged, persecuted, excessively sexual and with a dislike of restriction. Snakes hate constrictions; their neck is their weak point. They shed their skins, strike to kill, swallow things whole, etc.

Elaps Corallinus (Coral snake): black discharges; fear of rain; red spots in vision; green gung in nose; delusions and dreams of falling into an abyss. This snake hangs down from high places.

Cenchris (Copperhead snake): delusion in two places at
    once; right ovary, time passes slowly.

Crotalus Cascavella: warning rattle before striking.

Crotalus Horridus: decomposing (what happens when
    bitten).

Lachesis (Bush master, Surucucu snake): extrovert and
    entertaining; left-sided.

Naja Tripudians (Cobra): bitchy; pain from left ovary to
    heart (sex centre to heart).

Vipera (Common viper): bursting veins; worse leg hanging
    down; epigastrium pain.

Clotho Arictans (Puff adder): excessive puffy swelling.

Pelias Berus (Adder): navel pain (the umbilical cord is
    snake like).

Bungurus Fasciatus (Banded krait): acute myelitis; nerve
    sheath inflammation (snakes shed their skin).

A few homeopathic remedy pictures are described in more
detail as follows.

PULSATILLA

Pulsatilla types are people who need cuddles, company and
support. They are like the weeping willow tree, seemingly
unable to support any load, and look to strong partners for
support. They weep easily, yet they are not thirsty — an
interesting opposite. They tend to be plump and have soft
flesh — like they are soft and yielding inside. They use
manipulation to get their own way. They hate fat, and
prefer sweets, fade in the heat and stuffy rooms, often carry
fans, love fresh air, and slowly walking in it. In women,
menstrual periods tend to be short and their discharges
bland and yellow. They can become fanatical about a
subject once attached to it.

Phosphorous and Dolphin

These two are similar, embodying kindness, compassion, empathy, communication and love.

Phosphorous people are like the substance itself — as are all the remedy types. Phosphorus is the substance matchheads are made from; matches light up, burn brightly and go out, leaving dark remains. So these people exude kindness, compassion, openness, sensitive communication, but they do so to excess, burning out and getting sympathy exhaustion.

With treatment from the remedy *Phosphorus* they become more contained, and use their energy more wisely and effectively.

The *Dolphin* remedy is made from dolphin milk. Dolphins swim in the boundless sea, and are compassionate, kind creatures attracted to human company. They love to play and swim gracefully, and can also attack each other. In danger they move in circles around their young; the homeopathic provings show this feature — moving in circles, and the fear of outside attackers (sharks). People needing *Dolphin* suffer from internal dichotomies, as their great compassion can be over-stretched by the 'boundless seas'. Following treatment with the *Dolphin* remedy, however, they gain the strength to live without boundaries to their compassion.

There are subtle difference between these two remedies and their types; these can be seen here in the ability to cope with boundaries.

Dolphin and *Phosphorus*, for all their apparent differences in origin — fire and water — are similar in frequency or vibration. All healing professions (and physicists too) regard the body as a vibrating energetic pattern, rather than a fixed substance. We know that all the body systems, blood, lymph, brain fluid, nerves, digestion, etc. vibrate in a characteristic way. Although this is not yet scientifically proven, homeopaths believe that our remedies are complex vibrational patterns too.

SILICEA

Silicea types are like soft tanks — they yield to opposing forces such as domineering parents and teachers, but carry on in their own way just the same. They are stubborn, and concerned over small things. They become high achievers by persevering through lots of small steps to a substantial achievement. They fit the image of the perpetual student. A good academic or a thorough, meticulous achiever, they reach some recognised position where there is no component of overt aggression. Typical are maths and physics teachers and lecturers, electronic engineers and computer programmers — not those in business, politics or rough and tumble positions.

These people frequently have white spots on their finger nails, crippled toe nails, and are thin and chilly with smelly cold feet that embarrass them. They act timidly, with a discreet egotism; they lack the grit to face life, are refined and delicate, and do not argue. Once secure in a subject they can talk of nothing else, as they only feel safe to talk on well understood subjects. This is why they hate parties, which involve risks.

STRAMONIUM

Fear and terror predominate Stramonium types; their fear of violence sometimes turns into violent behaviour as a compensation for this fear. Most of their complaints are painless, and stuttering on the first word is a keynote indication that a person is of this type.

They have great fear of dogs, especially at night (dogs symbolise violence). They are also afraid of the dark, yet fascinated by it, and have a fear of water, of graves and churchyards, of coffins, and a fear of being alone at night, wanting instead light and company. Stramonium children have night terrors, and will sleep in their parents' bed. They are talkative, but this is confined to one subject.

They can be beseeching and religious, praying, or go into uncontrolled rage with increased strength — biting, hitting, strangling.

Stramonium is a good remedy for the fear following rape or other form of attack.

There are hundreds of other profiles and constitutional pictures. To illustrate the way in which a homeopathic remedy picture is built up, here is a detailed example below.

THUJA

Thuja is a wide ranging remedy suitable for constitutional prescribing, and for dealing with the deep miasmatic influences of gonorrhoea in the previous generations (resulting in growths, tumours, chronic sinusitis, chronic respiratory diseases, genital diseases and warts). It is also useful for antidoting the effects of vaccinations — especially the lifelong effects of smallpox vaccination — which are a recent cause of much chronic disease.

It is made from the bark of a tree that has usefulness in growing hedges. The hedge is a kind of barrier to the external world, and creating a barrier is a typical defence mechanism in Thuja people. These people are hidden behind a false image, created early in life. (Likewise a vaccination is meant to be a barrier to a disease.)

There are four levels to functioning as a person:
- self-confidence, which allows
- the ability to express oneself, which in turn allows
- the formation of boundaries in life (to say 'no' and mean it) which in turn allows
- effective living in the world.

Thuja people fall at the first hurdle. Self-confidence is something they did not get from their parenting. Instead an inner feeling of ugliness and frailty predominate, leading on to a great inability to communicate. They are secretive to an extreme, and give out very little about themselves at an interview or even to long-standing friends. They feel that others 'wouldn't like me if they knew me'.

Having virtually no ability to communicate means they cannot form adequate boundaries. Instead they try to fit in, to be accepted, not to stand out or be noticed, seek not to invite judgment or criticism in extreme, and are perfectionists in the social graces. They are superficially nice and charming — people pleasers — and are very conscious of the ego needs of others. Fitting in is their alternative to forming boundaries; this drives others to distraction, as when working with them they are like a chameleon, changing character and needs in relation to each and every person and situation. They are a moving mirror of who they are with, rather than people with their own unique expression.

Thuja people evolve a way of calculating how to fit in, withholding anything but the barest information needed in a situation — a sort of calculated deceit — about what they will let be known; they become compartmentalised, to an extreme degree.

BACKGROUND TO THUJA TYPES

Their childhood involved abuse, abandonment and emotional or physical neglect, where they received the idea that they were ugly, unlovable or bad. Encouragement was inadequate and punishment excessive — verbal or physical. This is internalised to create the belief that they have done something terribly wrong. They felt unhappy and tremendously lonely, but this may have happened at an age when they were too young to realise it. They feel deeply ashamed at being unwanted. From this comes the secrecy that makes a very poor boundary to the world. And from this backdrop develops a great inability to respond to others, hiding their true selves, creating a deep loneliness.

The achievements for which they may have been praised were their parents' goals, and so the idea of fitting in with others' expectations developed. They then gradually developed the appropriate character to avoid abuse and criticism; telling lies and withholding become essential elements of this approach. This becomes so routine that they no longer know what they want for themselves, nor who they are. They sculpture themselves in dress, cosmetics, gestures, posture, accent, even emotional expression. Their desire not to stand out, their pronounced invisibility, is a reliable guide to this type.

Inside, Thuja people feel not just ugly, but unlovable, full of guilt, unattractive whatever their appearance. Profoundly lonely, they are longing for a perfect mate, and find intimacy extraordinarily difficult. Outside they can become rigid, inflexible, brittle, ordered and very controlling.

In later life they can become fixed in their ideas, dogmatic and opinionated. They may become shy and reserved, or creative and imaginative, or haughty and incapable of small talk. This can lead on to alienation, isolation and extreme loneliness as they create a lifestyle reflecting their own inner drama of childhood, as we all do without fail. They may drift from one one-night-stand to another, from being heterosexual to gay, from one unfeeling situation to another. Because of their secretive nature they may develop into sneaky, evasive, furtive characters, or charming and captivating. From repeating failures to connect with others, and from being unable to express their emotions, they can get profoundly depressed, leading to successful suicides.

THUJA CHILDREN

They have fixed ideas and rigid self-made rules of behaviour; precocious and only relating to adults; affinity for music, pop, classical or church; very upset if they mess up their clothes by dropping food; won't go to parties; obsessed by fixed ideas about one thing or theme; rigidity of play; fear of strangers and touch by them; need delicate handling, feeling delicate and fragile inside; avoid physical games because of idea of fragility and injury; want to be carried rather than walk; mistrusting and believe others can listen in to their thoughts; stubborn about little things; tidy and meticulous.

KEYNOTE SYMPTOMS FOR THUJA PEOPLE

Worse from cold wet weather; virtually never worse from heat; worse on the left side; general improvement during a cold; worse 2–3 p.m., and 3 a.m. rarely; fragility, brittleness; a sensation of something alive in the abdomen; irritability only with their spouse where they feel secure; fastidious about the correct way to do something; deceitful, secretive, withholding; feels unattractive, ugly, unlovable; affinity for music, especially church music, and someone in the history who is associated with the church or church music; perspiration on uncovered parts; headache in the left temple, as if pierced by a nail at 3 a.m.; eyebrows are thin or lost on the outside; post natal discharge, thick; and chronic sinus problems; nasal polyps, worse left side; greasy, oily, waxy, shiny skin; old acne scars or cystic, hard acne, very common; warts and skin tags and tumours on face, eyelids, neck, body, hands, fingers, anus, soles; swallows words or speech trails off, uncommon but highly indicative; bulimic; intolerance of onions, flatulence after; desires sweets and chocolate (common symptoms); constipation with a hard stool; gonorrhoea past or present; herpes or venereal warts, on penis, vulva, vagina, cervix, anus; prostate enlargement and inflammation; inguinal glands swollen left side; strong sweetish odour of genitals; ovarian cysts, especially left-sided; uterine fibroids of all descriptions and polyps; chronic green thrush with fishy smell; deformed joints with little pain; deformed and brittle nails; sore soles making walking impossible in cold wet weather; chilblains and Raynaud's syndrome.

Caution: You may feel that you are at least partly a Thuja type of person. This is common, however, and no reason to try the remedy *Thuja*.

All homeopathic remedies overlap to a degree; the skill of the professional homeopath is to sort out the most appropriate remedy for each individual.

CHAPTER NINE

Case Studies

The case studies in this chapter show the diversity of homeopathy and its capacity to deal with a wide variety of problems. Each of the cases is genuine, and I have permission to use them.

CASE ONE: TOM

Tom is a mild, affectionate boy of fourteen who likes to be cuddled, and who wets his bed every night. He sleeps very deeply, and his parents cannot wake him up, presuming that this is due to his deep sleeping. They have tried the doctor and herbs to solve the problem, but to no effect.

TAKING THE CASE

Tom writes poems. He has a fear of spiders and the dark; has nightmares; likes to sleep with something to cuddle up to; is very sympathetic; likes animals a lot and has pets; and has very low self confidence. He is a very thirsty boy, and prefers salty food to sweets.

He gets very upset when told off, so upset that he goes to bed and stays there for quite a long time. He is almost ill, he is so sensitive. Tom can be quite witty and makes funny remarks, but only within the family — with strangers he is quite shy. He is good at humanities at school, but not the sciences. He has never had a close friend.

Tom was a small baby at birth, but otherwise the delivery was normal. There were no separations from his mother, and he was breast fed.

FAMILY BACKGROUND

Tom's mother is very anxious and fearful, quick tempered, and spoils the children a lot, fulfilling their every wish. His father is more of a hard, money seeking materialist. Tom has a younger brother who is quite different — insensitive, interested in money and business, with lots of confidence.

Tom's maternal grandfather died of a heart attack at around sixty; the other grandparents are all alive and have heart/circulation problems. Tom's father has high blood pressure, and has had a mild heart attack. There are no other diseases in the family.

This is a classic example of a very sensitive refined child with relatively insensitive parents. Tom gets upset and has symptoms from the stresses, fears and tensions common in a typical family.

REMEDY

Homeopathic *Phosphorus* was chosen on the signs of: mildness; reserved; liking cuddles and cuddling/clinging; fine features; fear of the dark; sympathetic; lack of confidence; love of animals; preference for humanities; likes chicken and salt; thirsty.

OUTCOME

Phosphorus was given originally, to great effect, and Tom's bed-wetting then happened only once a week. The family was delighted, but the homeopath felt that more could be done. Repetition of *Phosphorus* in a stronger dose helped further, and eighteen months after the first prescription his parents say Tom 'is a new boy'. He wets his bed occasionally.

CASE TWO: FRED

Fred is a man around thirty years old, who is confined to a wheelchair. This case is included to show how disease can develop.

TAKING THE CASE

Fred suffers mainly from cramps, spasms and convulsions, and an inability to control his muscles. While in company he stutters a lot, but not that much at home.

He is short-sighted and has nystagmus — oscillating eyeballs — and his vision is deteriorating. He is worried about losing his sight. Fred shakes on the least exertion, especially his hands, and gets cramps if he moves fast. He has to concentrate to get his muscles to obey his will, otherwise they won't do so. His stuttering is typical of this.

He gets electric-like feelings with bubbling sensations, like water out of a spring, that descend and flow down his body, with cramps and convulsions that start in his fingers. In convulsions he becomes unconscious, yet he can apparently still speak to people coherently. Also his lips go blue, and under his chin there is a blue line. The convulsions can come on from exertion, excitement, in sleep, from any conflict, evening and night, or from being moved.

He has a dry rash on his chest, which began fifteen years ago and first appeared behind his ears. It was treated with ointments from his doctor and went away, and shortly after that the convulsions started.

As a child, Fred was scared of being bullied, and played mostly with his younger brothers whom he looked after a lot. He is very nervous, and is scared of strangers. He cannot bear to go near the dentist's building, is nervous of noise and apprehensive about the future. He feels helpless.

Fred is happy to be with his brothers, and has no real friends. He has pleasant dreams of life at the time he was at school, and of red marks in his books. He is worse from heat, cold and sunlight. He used not to eat fruit and vegetables. He has whistling in his ears, sweats from fear and excitement and his eyelids are half open.

Two years ago he was given drugs at a hospital for the cramps, to reduce the copper imbalance he says, and after this he collapsed and has been in a wheelchair ever since.

Understanding this Situation

Fred stammered as a child, and was very fearful of bullying. From this I can presume two things: that he had a weak nervous system genetically, and that probably he was a slow child who got behind in his education (though this is a guess). His dreams of red marks in his books clearly imply being criticised; it may be that he was even hit at school or home for his presumed slowness, which would have affected him very badly, due to his sensitivity. As the first child it is likely that one parent at least was unskilled at parenting, and responded with reactions similar to what happened to them as a child — a very common phenomenon.

Fred is fearful of everything, so much so that he stays only with his brothers with whom he feels safe. Otherwise he finds the world a terrifying place, which he controls by being secluded in the family mesh.

The convulsions and cramps came on after the suppression of eruptions, which is a common medical error, and hospital treatment for copper imbalance apparently put him in a wheelchair. So this sensitive, nervous person has been very badly affected by his medical treatment. This, compounded by his early bad experiences

and original susceptibility, have combined to put him into
a wheelchair for life, unless something can be done to
reverse his state.

REMEDY

The essence of the case lies in his fears, suppression,
nervous disorders and convulsions.

After careful analysis, one of three homeopathic
remedies, *Gelsemium*, *Cuprum* or *Stramonium* will be the
choice.

The inner state of this man is critical to the final
decision — he seems to be someone who is very timid
and paralysed by fear.

> There are keynotes indications of Cuprum people —
> convulsions starting in the fingers, and the idea of
> being in charge in their own safe little world, inside a
> large world in which they perceive great danger.

On the other hand, *Stramonium* is strongly suggested for
fear of violence, bullies, that he talks about from
childhood. And Stramonium types stutter on the first
word, as Fred does, fighting to get control of his muscles.
However, his cowardice, fear of ordeals, anticipation, falling
eyelids, and the helpless paralysis which he is now in, hint
at *Gelsemium*.

On balance, it was thought that *Cuprum* would be the
best choice.

OUTCOME

Unfortunately, I do not know the outcome, as Fred is not
my patient. The prognosis is poor, however, because he is
already badly incapacitated and damaged nerves are hard to
heal — they may have suffered irreversible pathological
damage.

CASE THREE: TANIA — A CHILD OF CHERNOBYL

GENERAL BACKGROUND

Prior to Tania's birth, 1,000 metres up in the mountains of Bulgaria, there was a radioactive rain cloud from Chernobyl. A unique red rain was remembered, but no precautions taken as the people were not told about the nuclear disaster. In affected areas, leukaemia is one hundred times more common than it was prior to the disaster.

There was no history of any illness — including cancer — in this peasant family for three generations back. Yet at six years old, Tania developed cancer of the blood — leukaemia. The child got pains in her legs and a high fever, 39°C, in February 1993. She was given anti-fever medicine. The fever returned next day, and the dose was repeated.

Tania became so weak she could not walk. In hospital her condition was diagnosed as flu, for which she was given antibiotics. Blood tests were then done, and myeloblastic leukaemia diagnosed. Tania was given chemotherapy, radiation and cortisone treatment.

TAKING THE CASE

Tania was seen under very difficult conditions, with sceptical parents, through translators with insufficient time and difficult follow-ups.

I observed that Tania has very long eyelashes. While sleeping she weeps and screams, dreaming about sports cars that run her over; she is hard to wake up; used to sleep on her front.

There is some conflict with a sister who is two years younger. Tania is jealous and weepy when not the centre of attention; weeps from trifles; very helpful child; only had chicken pox before serious illness (the only childhood disease for which she was not vaccinated).

Tania likes sweets and especially chocolate; not fond of meat or fat; likes soft-boiled eggs; loves vinegar; likes green vegetables and bananas; not thirsty.

She prefers company of her mother and to entertain smaller children — takes them for walks.

Since being ill, Tania has been capricious, wild, hitting the wall, tearing her skin and picking her lips. She touches her genitals a lot, and has done all her life.

Chemotherapy does not seem to affect her except that her hair has fallen out; plays as normal. She likes the sun.

REMEDY

Tania was given homeopathic *Pulsatilla*, LM1, from 5 July 1993 for twenty-four days.

OUTCOME

Afterwards Tania was much more lively, and happy to be at home. For the first night she could not sleep and needed to wee frequently (something she had not experienced before), and for one night she had a high fever — 39°C. There were, however, no great changes in her condition.

Tania relapsed after a blood transfusion and cytotoxic drugs (to destroy malignant cells). She had a periodic high fever (39°C). There was blood in her urine, and she was not thirsty.

Because she had no hair, Tania's friends made fun of her, which offended her; she dreams of offence; sensitive to insult; picks fights with her sister — the butt of her anger — and destroys her sister's games. Indifferent to her sister; indifferent to consolation; capricious; wants mother for herself; detached, sad and apathetic.

IMPORTANT BACKGROUND EMERGES

One day Tania's father came home very pent-up. He threw his wife's belongings out the door, shouted at and started to beat her. He broke two of her teeth and gave her black eyes in this violent attack, during which he threatened to kill her. She grabbed Tania and ran, but he chased them. There was a series of violent exchanges, until finally she escaped and hid all night under a nearby building.

Tania witnessed all this, and since then has not let her father near her mother.

After the crisis Tania suddenly became ill. The lowering of Tania's immunity created by the family trauma allowed the radiation induced leukaemia to get established. Medical research has indicated that emotional trauma depresses the immune system, and that any disease process waiting in the wings can then develop.

The violent episode was discussed, and once the father appreciated its potentially dire consequences, he also participated. His daughter's life was more important to him than admitting to violent behaviour. This conversation must have acted as a focus for resolving at least some of the damage.

SECOND REMEDY

I prescribed *Sepia*, LM1, in September 1993.

OUTCOME

Tania's blood tests returned rapidly to normal, and she had no more blood transfusions. She has remained this way for over two years to date. The hospital consultants were reportedly very surprised at the speed of her recovery.

CONCLUSION

Discussing the family crisis openly, and its resolution, must have helped Tania. Her case shows the potency of the homeopathic approach even in very difficult and apparently hopeless cases — cure the effects of the underlying trauma; release the immune depression; and the body's natural defences will do the rest.

The way homeopaths see illnesses such as cancer and diabetes is as follows. We all have disease processes lurking in the wings, but our natural immune system is dealing with these all the time; removing cancer cells or restricting diabetic development is a normal, constant process.

> An emotional or physical shock to the system can block the energy flow, and immunity can fall. If it falls below a critical point in the person, the most prominent latent disease takes hold.

CASE FOUR: ANNA

Anna is a teacher, and she is married with one son. She has had epilepsy since the age of fourteen, with both petit mals (little fits) and grand mals (big fits).

BACKGROUND

Following her pregnancy and because she tried not taking her medicine, Anna's fits returned. She has since had three miscarriages, at four, two and three months gestation — no reasons were found; she had a stitch to hold the second living child in the uterus.

Anna has problems in her relationship with her husband, and has tried to divorce him three times; she changes her mind, as he threatens to kill himself. Her feelings about divorce are contradictory — she wants to do it, but is fearful of being alone. She always wants to be with her friends, as she cannot be alone, but her husband is very jealous of them, so this is difficult. At one point she had several affairs as a protest.

Anna likes her teaching job in a kindergarten (I see her as childish). She also enjoys physical activity such as gymnastics — it calms her. If she is depressed, going to the mountains helps. She is into spiritual meditation, which helps too. Before joining a spiritual group she used to cry a lot.

Anna has made two attempts at suicide. She takes pills, then calls the ambulance as she thinks of her child. The first attempt happened because her situation with her husband was so hopeless, the second after being reprimanded by the headmaster where she teaches.

ANNA'S FITS

Prior to a fit, Anna begins moaning, and has palpitations. Her right arm goes stiff, and she drops anything she may be carrying. It starts in the solar plexus, and then goes to the head. She has a mocking inner voice when an epileptic attack is about to happen, and voices sound as if on a slow tape winding down to a stop. Everything goes in slow motion. She tries to calm herself down, but to no avail.

During an attack (they are left-sided) she gets a nervous crisis and uneven heartbeat. She feels tired, her eyes are open and she loses consciousness. She mumbles and moans. Afterwards, Anna feels confused.

She has grand mals about twice a year, and at night only; petit mals can be in the daytime. An electrocardiogram (ECG) did not show anything.

TAKING THE CASE

Anna is in despair over her marriage — she can't live with her husband, but nor can she leave him.

Her recent periods have been twenty-one and ten days long. She is a hot person, uncovers her feet at night; desires fresh air; likes spring; wakes between 3 and 4 a.m. since breast feeding. Desires fruit and chocolate; not thirsty; sighs with a lump in the throat.

Anna can't cry and is averse to consolation, and to the sun. Music makes her feel better.

Headaches (often left-sided) are better from tight binding; before her period; worse from sun.

She hates cats. She dwells on past disagreeable occurrences; has burning enthusiasms which evaporate. When she is upset, everything becomes unreal and gets very bright. A fuse goes inside her, and she cannot help shouting and quarrelling. Calmness is a big issue for her.

Anna feels chilly before menses; feels unfortunate; frowns. Everything shows on her face. There is some confusion in her head.

She has had a crusty head eruption with white scales, since the age of eleven. It has been suppressed by ointments, preceding onset of fits.

REMEDY

Cicuta was the remedy indicated, and I gave Anna one dose. *Cicuta* was chosen after two other remedies failed to cure. It was based on epilepsy brought on by suppression of eruptions, her childish nature, and many specific peculiarities of her symptoms.

OUTCOME

Anna became more decisive and more resolute. She decided finally to divorce her husband — this time no one can persuade her to do otherwise. Everyone says she is a new woman — younger, sunnier, more beautiful and youthful. Whereas before she quarrelled over many things, she is now wiser (a change in awareness). Anna is now more wilful, having previously been indecisive and suggestible. She is much calmer when speaking, and more coherent.

The eruption on her head returned, and is now disappearing. The symptom she had prior to having epilepsy — cheek numbness — has returned.
Anna has had no grand mals for a year and her petit mals have reduced very significantly.

CONCLUSION

Curing epilepsy is not so difficult, but the management of the cure is. For example, a car driver cannot stop taking the drugs, because if she has a fit while driving it is not only dangerous but she will also lose her licence. Most people are also very concerned — often needlessly — about the damage caused by a fit. In addition, the drugs can prevent a homeopath from being able to understand the case fully. It is best to try to cure epilepsy as soon as it occurs, and not wait for many years of drug suppression.

Helpful Addresses

UNITED KINGDOM

To find a homeopathic practitioner in your area, or for your nearest homeopathic pharmacy, contact the following organisations:

The British Homeopathic Association

27a Devonshire Street, London W1N 1RJ.
Tel.: 0171 935 2163.

(For a list of doctors who practise homeopathy.)

The Society of Homeopaths

2 Artizan Road, Northampton NN1 4HU.
Tel.: 01604 21400.

(The Society of Homeopaths has a register of professional homeopaths.)

If you are considering training in homeopathy, consult the Society of Homeopaths above for a list of recommended colleges.

Doctors who wish to train in homeopathy can consult:

The Faculty of Homeopathy

Royal London Homeopathic Hospital, Great Ormond Street, London WC1N 1HR.
Tel.: 0171 837 3091, ext. 7285.

The Oxford Course

Homeopathic Physicians Teaching Group, 28 Beaumont Street, Oxford OX1 2NP.

Those interested in research can contact:

The Homeopathic Trust for Research and Education

2 Powis Place, London WC1N 3HT.
Tel.: 0171 837 9469; Fax: 0171 278 7900.

IRELAND

Herbal and Homeopathic Clinic
Halmont Ltd, Eagle House, Sidmonton Avenue, Bray,
Co. Wicklow. Tel.: 01 286 6280.

The Irish Medical Homeopathic Association
32 Upper Baggot Street, Dublin 4. Tel.: 01 668 3996.

The Irish Society of Homeopaths
66 Mount Anville Wood, Dublin 14. Tel.: 01 288 6344.

Morehampton Pharmacy
79 Morehampton Road, Dublin 4. Tel.: 01 668 7103.

Nelson's Pharmacy
15 Duke Street, Dublin 2. Tel.: 01 679 0451.

HOMEOPATHIC PHARMACIES

*Most chemists and healthfood shops stock a limited range of
homeopathic remedies. For the full range of remedies, however, a
specialised pharmacy is required. All products can be supplied by
post urgently if requested.*

Ainsworths
36 Cavendish Street, London W1M 7LH.
Tel.: 0171 935 5330; Fax: 0171 486 4313.

Buxton & Grant
176 Whiteladies Road, Bristol BS8 2XU.
Tel.: 01272 735025.

Freeman's Pharmacy
7 Eaglesham Road, Clarkston, Glasgow G76 7BU.
Tel.: 0141 644 1165.

Galen Homeopathic
Lewell Mill, West Stafford, Dorchester, Dorset DT2 8AN.
Tel.: 01305 263996.

Goulds
14 Crowndale Road, London NW1 1TT.
Tel.: 0171 388 4752.

Helios

97 Camden Road, Tunbridge Wells, Kent TN1 2QR.
Tel.: 01892 536393; Fax: 01892 546850.

Nelson's Homeopathic Pharmacy

73 Duke Street, London W1M 6BY. Tel.: 0171 629 3118.

Phials, storage boxes, unmedicated tablets and other homeopathic supplies, charts etc., and a catalogue of such products (no remedies, however) can be obtained from:

The Homeopathic Supply Co.

4 Nelson Road, Sheringham, Norfolk NR26 8BU.
Tel.: 01263 824683.

Complaints Index

Recommended Reading

A catalogue of homeopathic books is available from:
Minerva Books, 6 Bothwell Street, London W6 8DY.
Tel./Fax: 0181 385 0861.

You may also wish to read the following:

Chappell, Peter, *Emotional Healing with Homeopathy*, London:
Element Books 1994.

Castro, Miranda, *The Complete Handbook of Homeopathy*,
London: Macmillan 1989. (A very detailed book, full of
useful, practical information.)

Handley, Rima, *A Homeopathic Love Story*, USA: North
Atlantic Books 1990. (An excellent historical book.)

Herscu, Paul, *The Homeopathic Treatment of Children*, USA:
North Atlantic Books 1991.

Lessell, Dr Colin, *The World Traveller's Manual of Homeopathy*,
Saffron Walden: CW Daniel 1993.

Sheppard, Dr Dorothy, *Homeopathy for the First Aider*, Saffron
Walden: CW Daniel 1945. (An often reprinted classic.)

Whitmont, Edward, *Alchemy of Healing*, USA: North
Atlantic Books 1993. (A real psychological gem.)

The following books are for practising homeopaths:

Morrison, Roger, *The Desk Top Prescriber*, USA: Hahnemann
Clinic Publishing 1993. (One of my favourites for
professional use.)

Vermeulin, Frans, *Concordant Materia Medica*, Holland:
Merlin Publishers 1994. (The best composite *materia
medica* so far.)

Vithoulkas, George, *The Science of Homeopathy*, London:
Thorsons 1980. (This is the best text book available on
homeopathy.)

The following two books are the best repertories available:

Schroyens, Frederik, *The Synthesis Repertory*, Belgium:
Homeopathic Books 1995.

Zandvoort, Roger van, *The Complete Repertory of the Mind*,
Holland: Institute for Research in Homeopathic
Information and Symptomatology 1994.

Note:

Peter Chappell cannot enter into correspondence about any illness
or disease. If you have other queries, please send a letter with a
stamped addressed envelope if you wish to receive a reply, to:
The Stanlake Practice, 5a Stanlake Rd, London W12 7HE.
You may fax or email Peter Chappell on:
Fax +44 181 749 0093; email: peterchappel@gn.apc.org

Index